ACKNOWLEDGEMENTS

My obligations to individuals and institutions who contributed to the publication of this book are numerous, and only partially discharged by this brief expression of appreciation.

Special thanks go to my colleagues past and present who have co-authored many of the concepts contained in this book: Nichols Vorys, M.D.; Paige Besch, Ph.D.; Clyde H. Dorr II, M.D.; Sergio Stone, M.D.; Jane Weems Chihal, M.D., Ph.D.; Richard Peppler, Ph.D.; Steven N. Taylor, M.D.; Phillip H. Rye, M.D.; Peter Lu, M.D.; and especially Louise B. Tyrer, M.D. for her contribution of the section "Teenagers and OCs."

Thanks also go to my office manager Susie White, the rest of the staff of the Fertility Institute of New Orleans and to Lynda Blake, Desmond Bond, and the staff of EMIS, Inc.

A very special thanks goes to readers whose suggestions have been incorporated to improve the accuracy and usefulness of this book.

DEDICATION

To Dr. John Wells, co-founder of Creative Infomatics (now EMIS, Inc.), who first adapted the center index format for use in a medical publication and whose collaboration made this effort possible to improve patient care.

TABLE OF CONTENTS

TABLES

PREFACE

New oral contraceptive (OC) formulations, new and better ways of using OCs, and new methods of hormonal contraception, continue to be discovered some 40 years after introduction of the first OC, Enovid® in 1960. A clinical study, 35 years ago[1], formed the basis for *Managing Contraceptive Pill Patients* (*MCPP*); the 1st edition, published 27 years ago, was guided by a number of additional sources[2]. The need continues for up-to-date, accurate information about OCs and other forms of hormonal contraception, their beneficial and adverse effects, and the management of women using hormonal contraception.

The 12th edition of *MCPP* contains changes to make using the guide easier to use, including:

- The Center Index has been revised;
- References have been placed at the end of each section and table instead of being listed in a single block at the end of the book. Numerous new references have been added;
- The contraceptive hormone vaginal ring, transdermal patch, and IUDs, each have their own section;
- Table 3: Pregnancy and Continuation Rates, has been included;
- The Inactive Ingredients listed in Table 5 have been enhanced and reorganized;
- Section 12: Emergency Contraception and parts of other sections have been expanded.
- An enhanced Index.

Since the 11th edition, some OC labels have been discontinued, or are being distributed by different manufacturers. At least twelve new labels have been added, and one new oral contraceptive formulation, Seasonale®, has been introduced. Seasonale® is the first 'Extended-Cycle' OC, in which active combination pills are taken continuously for 84 days followed by 7 days of rest or inactive pills, and results in nine additional weeks of OC use during a calendar year. Only one extended cycle OC is presently available in the US.

The 11th edition of *MCPP* coincided with the introduction of three new progestins: drospirenone, etonogestrel and norelgestromin. Two totally new oral contraceptive pill formulations—Cyclessa® a desogestrel based triphasic pill, and Yasmin®, a drospirenone-based combination pill—were added. Also, three new hormonal contraceptive devices, namely NuvaRing® a vaginal ring, Ortho-Evra® a transdermal contraceptive patch, and Mirena® a levonorgestrel-loaded intrauterine contraceptive device (IUD), were introduced. Drospirenone is an analogue of spironolactone, with antimineralocorticoid and antiandrogenic activity; Etonogestrel (3-keto-desogestrel) is the progestin component of the biologically active metabolite of desogestrel; Norelgestromin (levonorgestrel-3-oxime) is the progestin component of the primary serum metabolite of norgestimate. A third new OC formulation, Ortho Tri-Cyclen® LO, was added in the third printing of the 11th edition.

The second and third printings of the 10th edition of *MCPP* added information about Lunelle® (a once-per-month contraceptive injection) and about Mifeprex® (mifepristone, RU 486) which had received FDA approval. Since the 11th edition, distribution of both Lunelle® and Mifeprex® has been suspended.

Following the 9th edition, the length of the text was reduced by removing redundant or out-of-date information and many superceded references, most notably in the sections on the cardiovascular system, the breast, and effects of OCs on pregnancy. A reader who is interested in this older information may contact us.

Since the 1st edition, published in 1977, *MCPP* has introduced many concepts concerning oral contraceptive use that have become part of the U.S. FDA's required package insert. They include

- the use of the lowest doses of estrogen and progestin consistent with effectiveness;
- that the net effect of an OC depends on the type and/or amount of progestin, and on a balance between the estrogen and progestin components;

- a listing of the benefits of OC use; and
- information about the relationship of estrogen to cardiovascular disease.

The "Pill Book" remains the only single source of information about real differences between OCs in estrogenic, androgenic, progestational, and endometrial (breakthrough bleeding) potencies, and regarding management of side effects in relation to these differences.

Readers are invited to send suggestions for changes and new information they believe should be included in *Managing Contraceptive Pill Patients* to the author, care of the publisher, by e-mail at http://www.emispub.com, or by fax to (214) 495-8530. If the information is used, the sender will receive a free copy of the next printing of *MCPP*. As always, new information is added to each new printing.

R.P.D.
New Orleans
June 2004

1. Dickey RP, Dorr CH II: Oral Contraceptives: Selection of the Proper Pill. Obstet Gynecol 1969;33:273
2. Studies at Louisiana State University (including Chihal HJW, Dickey RP, Peppler R: Estrogen Potency of Oral Contraceptive Pills, Am J Obstet Gynecol 1975;121:75–83, and Dickey RP: The Pill: Physiology, Pharmacology, and Clinical Use, in: *Seminar in Family Planning*, 1st ed. Isenman AW, Knox EG, Tyrer L (eds.) American College of Obstetrics and Gynecology, 1972; 2nd ed., 1974) and in the Philippines (see Wells JP, Dickey RP, Porter CW: Report of the Survey Team Concerning the Decrease in Pill Acceptors in the Phillipines Family Planning Program, March 22, 1973. American Public Health Association, 1015 18th Street NW, Washington, D.C. 20036.).

INTRODUCTION

Popularity of OC Use

Oral contraceptives (OCs) are the most widely used and successful method of reversible birth control in the world. Since their introduction in 1960, the acceptance and popularity of OCs have continued due to their:

- High rate of effectiveness
- Simple method of use
- Ease of discontinuance
- Rapid reversal of effects after discontinuance
- Beneficial effects on the menstrual cycle.

Risks of OC Use

The risks associated with OC use (see Table 2) are low compared to the risk to life associated with pregnancy, except in women who:

- Smoke cigarettes and are older than age 35
- Have Leiden factor V mutation (1).

Reducing Risks

Nearly all the excess risk of death due to OC use can be attributed to cardiovascular disease. The increased risk of cardiovascular disease may continue for a number of years after OCs are stopped. Both long- and short-term risks may be reduced if women:

- Use OCs containing smaller and less biologically active amounts of estrogen and progestin
- Are carefully screened, and those at high risk advised to choose other contraceptive methods
- Recognize and report clinical symptoms that may precede serious illness early in their occurrence.

Health personnel are often faced with the dilemma of choosing between an OC with high hormone activity in order to ensure regular menses and continued patient use and an OC with low hormone activity in order to reduce side effects. The choice of OC must be individualized for each patient.

OC Patient Management

The essential elements for good management of OC patients are:

- Knowledge of the contraindications to OC use, both absolute and relative (see Section 8)
- Knowledge of the causes of common side effects (see Section 5)
- The ability to recognize potentially serious illnesses as soon as they occur (see Table 11)
- Access to accurate information about biological activity differences among OCs (see Section 4).

Using This Text

Clinical information about the frequency of most of the known OC side effects and their usual outcomes is provided in this text as well as a recommended plan of their management. In many cases, the recommended course of management is to switch patients to OCs with different levels of one of the four major biological activities. Table 6 lists these categorical activities and should prove helpful to clinicians as they choose OCs.

The activity profiles of various OCs are especially advantageous for the selection of an initial OC (see Section 11). The number of women who can successfully use OCs can be increased if the initial OC is selected to avoid particular side effects. Patients can later be switched to different OC formulations (determined according to their biological activity rankings) if side effects occur.

Recommendations for selecting an initial OC are summarized in Table 8. OCs listed in Table 9 are categorized into 13 groups according to their estrogen amounts and progestational, androgenic, and endometrial activities. OCs from Groups 1, 2, 5 to 8, and 10 have 35 mcg or less estrogen and the lowest androgen activities. OCs in these groups may reduce immediate and delayed cardiovascular side effects.

Approximately 90% of patients should be able to take at least one of the OCs containing less than 35 mcg estrogen without experiencing symptoms of menstrual irregularity after the third cycle of use.

References for Introduction

1. Vandenbrouke JP, Koster T, Briet E, et al.: Increased risk of venous thrombosis in oral contraceptive users who are carriers of factor V Leiden mutation. Lancet 1994;344:1453–1457.

SECTION 1: BENEFITS OF OCs TO REPRODUCTIVE HEALTH

Benefits of OC Use

Women receive significant benefits during and after discontinuing OC use (see Table 1). These benefits include:

- Avoidance of pregnancy-related complications (1)
- Reduced premenstrual symptoms and menstruation-related anemia. (2, 3, 4)
- Reduced incidence of endometrial and ovarian cancers (5, 6, 7, 8, 9, 10, 11, 12, 13)
- Reduced incidence of gynecological diseases that cause infertility (2, 14, 15, 16)
- Reduced incidence of colorectal cancer (17, 18).

It is estimated that, for every 100,000 OC users, the following pregnancy-related conditions (19) are avoided:

- 117 ectopic pregnancies
- 10,500 spontaneous abortions
- 10,407 term pregnancies requiring Cesarean sections.

Complications of these conditions are the leading causes of maternal deaths in young women.

Additionally, breast biopsies are reduced in OC users (1, 20, 21, 22).

An important beneficial effect of OCs for women who want to delay child-bearing is the protection provided against four of the most frequent causes of infertility:

- Endometriosis (2, 14, 16)
- Pelvic inflammatory disease (PID) (15)
- Ovarian cysts (3, 14, 23)
- Uterine fibroids (2, 14).

These diseases account for approximately 50% of all infertility due to a female factor and 90% of infertility that requires surgical treatment.

MANAGING

CONTRACEPTIVE

PILL PATIENTS

Twelfth Edition

by Richard P. Dickey, MD, PhD
(Pharmacology)

Chairman, Medical Advisory Board, Louisiana State
Family Planning Program; F.A.C.O.G.;
Board Certified Obstetrics and Gynecology,
Board Certified Reproductive Endocrinology and Infertility;
Clinical Professor of Obstetrics and Gynecology, and
Chief Section of Reproductive Endocrinology and Infertility,
Louisiana State University School of Medicine, New Orleans;
Medical Director, The Fertility Institute of New Orleans.

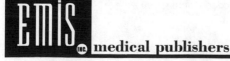
EMIS, INC. medical publishers

Direct Mail Orders
EMIS, Inc.
P.O. Box 820062
Dallas, TX 75382-0062

Telephone Orders
1-800-225-0694

FAX Your Order
(214) 495-8530

E-Mail Your Order
http://www.emispub.com

MANAGING CONTRACEPTIVE PILL PATIENTS
Twelfth Edition

ISBN 0-917634-31-4

Published in the United States 2004

First Edition 1977
Second Edition 1980
Third Edition 1983
Fourth Edition 1984
Fifth Edition 1987
Sixth Edition 1991
Seventh Edition 1993
Eighth Edition 1994
Ninth Edition 1998
Tenth Edition 2000
Second Printing 2001
Third Printing 2001
Eleventh Edition 2002
Second Printing 2002
Third Printing 2003
Twelfth Edition 2004
Second Printing 2004

This text is printed on recycled paper

Safety of Use

Combination OCs are equal to or surpass other contraceptive methods in safety compared to pregnancy until age 35 for smokers and throughout life for nonsmokers (see Table 2) (24, 25, 26, 27, 28). To minimize risks, older women should be cautioned to take the lowest dose formulation that maintains menstrual regularity.

All of the increased mortality associated with OC use is related to cardiovascular disease (CVD). OC use is safe throughout reproductive life in women who:

1. Have no cardiovascular risk factors, i.e.:
   - Hypertension
   - Obesity
   - Hyperlipidemia
2. Have no family history of CVD
3. Do not smoke
4. Use regimens containing an average estrogen dose of less than 50 mcg
5. Do not have Leiden factor V mutation (29).

A further reduction of the hazards of combination OCs may be achieved with:
- Progestin-only OCs
- Progestin injections
- Progestin implants
- Progestin-containing IUDs
- OCs with progestational and androgenic potencies less than or equal to 0.5 mg of norethindrone.

References for Section 1: Benefits of OCs to Reproductive Health

1. Ory HW: The noncontraceptive health benefits from oral contraceptive use. Fam Plann Perspect 1982;14:182.
2. Royal College of General Practitioners. Oral contraceptives and health: An interim report from the oral contraception study of the Royal College of General Practitioners. New York: Pitman, 1974.
3. Vessey MP et al.: A long-term follow-up study of women using different methods of contraception: An interim report. J Biosoc Sci 1976;8:373–427.

4. Walnut Creek Contraceptive Drug Study. Results of the Walnut Creek Contraceptive Drug Study. J Repro Med 1980;25(suppl):346.

5. Centers for Disease Control Cancer and Steroid Hormone Study. Oral contraceptive use and the risk of ovarian cancer. JAMA 1983;249:1596–1599.

6. Cohen CJ, Deppe G: Endometrial carcinoma and oral contraceptive pills. Am J Obstet Gynecol 1977;49:390–392.

7. Kaufman DW et al.: Decreased risk of endometrial cancer among oral contraceptive users. N Engl J Med 1980;303:1045.

8. Kay CR: Progestogens before and after menopause. Br Med J 1980;281:811–812.

9. Scotlenfeld D, Engle RL Jr: Decreased risk of endometrial cancer among oral contraceptive users. N Engl J Med 1980;303:1045.

10. Silverberg SG, Makowski EL: Endometrial carcinoma in young women taking oral contraceptive agents. Am J Obstet Gyencol 1975;46:503–506.

11. Silverberg SG, Makowski EL, Roche WD: Endometrial carcinoma in women under 40 years of age: Comparisons of cases in oral contraceptive users and nonusers. Cancer 1977;39:592–598.

12. Weiss NS et al.: Incidence of ovarian cancer in relation to use of oral contraceptives. Int J Cancer 1981;28:669–671.

13. Weiss NS, Sayvetz TA et al.: Incidence of endometrial cancer in relation to oral contraceptives. N Engl J Med 1980;302:551.

14. Chiaffarino Francesca et al.: Oral contraceptive use and benign gynecologic conditions. Contraception 1998;57:11–18.

15. Senanayake P, Kramer DG: Contraception and the etiology of PID: New perspectives. Am J Obstet Gynecol 1980;138:852–860.

16. Vessey MP, Villard-MacKintosh L, Painter R: Epidemiology of endometriosis in women attending family planning clinics. Br Med J 1993;306:182–184.

17. Fernandez E, La Vecchia C, Balducci A, Chatenoud L, Franceschi S, Negri E. Oral contraceptives and colorectal cancer risk: a meta analysis. Br J Cancer 2001;84:722–7.

18. Fernandez E, La Vecchia C, Franceschi S, Braga C, Talamini R, Negri E, Parazzini F. Oral contraceptives use and risk of colorectal cancer risk. Epidemiology 1998;9:295–300.

19. Petitti D, Wingerd J: Use of oral contraceptives, cigarette smoking, and risk of subarachnoid hemorrhage. Lancet 1978;2:234–236.

20. Ory HW: Oral contraceptive use and breast diseases. In: Pharmacology of Steroid Contraceptive Drugs. Garattini S, Berendes HW (ed.) New York: Raven Press, 1977;179–183.

21. Ory HW et al.: Oral contraceptives and reduced risk of benign breast diseases. N Engl J Med 1976;294:419–422.

4

22. Royal College of General Practitioners Oral Contraceptive Study. Effect on hypertension and benign breast disease of progestogen component in combined oral contraceptives. Lancet 1977;1:624.

23. Ylikorkala O: Ovarian cysts and hormonal contraception. Lancet 1977;1:1101–1102.

24. Porter JB et al.: Oral contraceptives and nonfatal vascular disease. Obstet Gynecol 1985;66:1–4.

25. Porter JB, Hershel J, Walker AM: Mortality among oral contraceptive users. Obstet Gynecol 1987;70:29–32.

26. Tietze C: New estimates of mortality associated with fertility control. Fam Plann Perspect 1977; 9(2):74–76.

27. Trussell J, Hatcher RA, Cates W Jr., Stewart FH, Kost K: A guide to interpreting contraceptive efficacy studies. Obstet Gynecol 1990;76:558–567.

28. Trussell J, Kost K: Contraceptive failure in the United States: A critical review of the literature. Stud Fam Plann1987;18(5):237–283.

29. Vandenbrouke JP, Koster T, Briet E, et al.: Increased risk of venous thrombosis in oral contraceptive users who are carriers of factor V Leiden mutation. Lancet 1994;344:1453–1457.

SECTION 2: THERAPEUTIC USES
OF OCs

Dysfunctional Uterine Bleeding

OCs may be used in the treatment of dysfunctional uterine bleeding (DUB) not due to organic causes.

DUB is common at the beginning and end of reproductive life but may occur throughout reproductive life in some women. DUB may result from anovulatory cycles or inadequate production of estrogen or progesterone. Treatment of nearly all forms of DUB can be accomplished with a balanced OC that has high endometrial activity (see Table 6). Some cases may also be treated with triphasic OCs.

Dysmenorrhea

See Section 21.

Endometriosis and Adenomyosis

High-dose OCs are no longer recommended for treatment of endometriosis. OCs with low estrogen doses are recommended for long-term management to delay recurrence of disease, especially when preservation of fertility is desired. The severity of endometriosis is reduced and the time until remission may be increased by low-estrogenic/high-progestational activity OCs because these decrease the amount of menstrual flow and block ovulation (1, 2, 3). Epidemiological studies show that current use of OCs has a significant protective effect (relative risk [RR] = 0.4) against endometriosis (3). However, this effect may not persist in former users (1).

Some clinicians advocate taking three packets of OCs (63 pills) consecutively in order to decrease the number of menstrual days (4). The availability of extended cycle regimens (Seasonale®) makes this easier to accomplish. However, the number of bleeding days is not decreased in extended cycle regimens, compared to 28-day regimens, for all patients. Women with endometriosis should continue OC use until the cycle preceding the one in which they intend to become pregnant.

Polycystic Ovaries

OCs may be used in the treatment of polycystic ovary syndrome (PCOS) (Stein-Leventhal syndrome) to suppress androgenic effects and prevent endometrial cancer by induction of regular withdrawal bleeding.

PCOS is characterized by excessive androgen effects (hair growth, acne, obesity, and irregular menses). Other conditions that present identical signs and symptoms are:

- Insulin resistance
- Ovarian hyperthecosis
- Ovarian stromal hyperplasia
- Ovarian and/or adrenal neoplasia
- Late onset adrenogenital syndrome
- Cushing's syndrome.

These conditions are all characterized by excessive production of biologically active androgens and frequently are improved by OC use. Excessive amounts of androgen produced in the ovaries are suppressed by the progestin component of the OC, while the sex hormone-binding globulin (SHBG) production is increased by the estrogen component. When estrogen levels are low, the amount of free testosterone increases relative to the amount of bound testosterone. Thus, clinical relief of androgen symptoms will likely occur when a moderate or high estrogen OC is taken, even though the production rate of androgen is unchanged. This positive effect of OCs is further enhanced when the estrogen is combined with a progestin that has low androgenic but high progestational activity, such as desogestrel or ethynodiol diacetate (5, 6).

It is important that a diagnosis be established before beginning treatment. Fasting insulin and blood glucose levels should be performed, since 40% of PCOS patients will be found to have insulin resistance. Pelvic ultrasound and DHEAS should be performed to rule out neoplasia and adrenal causes of excessive androgen.

Once a diagnosis is established, excessive androgen production of ovarian origin can be suppressed with combination OCs that have high progestational and low androgenic activities (see Table 9, Groups 2, 6, and 10).

Decreased sebum production can usually be seen within one cycle of OC use. A patient's failure to improve within this time is an indication that excess androgen may not be of ovarian origin. Patients with hyperthecosis or stromal hyperplasia, however, usually require longer treatment periods for suppression of ovarian activity and may not achieve such suppression at all. Suppression of hair growth requires more lengthy treatment; reversal of abnormal hair growth may not be apparent for many months.

Acne Vulgaris

See Section 34.

Ovarian Dysgenesis

Ovarian dysgenesis (primary ovarian failure or Turner's syndrome, XO karyotype) is characterized by failure to develop secondary sex characteristics. A diagnosis of ovarian dysgenesis should be established by chromosomal analysis. Other causes of failure to develop sex characteristics or menstruate include pituitary and ovarian tumors.

When height growth has ceased, significant psychological benefits may be achieved by stimulation of secondary sex characteristics and/or menses with estrogen. When maximum breast development has been achieved or menstrual spotting or bleeding occurs, the patient can be switched to a sub-50 mcg estrogen combination or multiphasic OC to reduce the risk associated with unopposed estrogen.

Premature Menopause

Premature menopause (secondary ovarian failure) may be treated with either estrogen replacement therapy or low-dose OCs that have a neutral effect on serum lipids. OCs are especially indicated for women younger than age 35.

Hormone replacement treatment should only be started for these women after the diagnosis is confirmed by high levels of follicle-stimulating hormone (FSH). Because of occasional remission in spontaneous premature menopause, some clinicians discontinue hormone annually for six weeks in order to determine if spontaneous menses will resume.

Menopause

To replace ovarian hormones lost at menopause completely, progesterone and androgen are necessary in addition to estrogen because ovaries produce all three types of hormones during reproductive years. Low-dose estrogen OCs meet this criterion and may be used instead of estrogen alone if serum lipid levels are normal and patients do not smoke cigarettes. In addition, combination OCs may decrease the possibility of endometrial and ovarian cancers (7, 8). OCs containing 20 mcg or higher EE amounts provide higher estrogenic activities than are ordinarily used for hormonal replacement therapy (HRT); 10 mcg of EE is approximately equivalent to 1 mcg of micronized estradiol or 0.625 mcg of conjugated equine estrogen when taken orally.

Blood Dyscrasia

Low-dose OCs have been used in cases of blood dyscrasia, when it is desirable to reduce the amount of menstrual flow. An alternative method of hormonal treatment is the repeated injection of MPA in doses of 100 mg every two weeks. Treatment intervals and doses of MPA may be increased to 150 mg every three months or to 400 mg every six months. Continuous spotting may occur in up to 50% of patients during the first six months of MPA use.

Amenorrhea Pregnancy Testing

OCs have no place in the evaluation of amenorrhea or as a test for pregnancy. Instead, if the duration of amenorrhea is less than 10 weeks, 50 mg progesterone in oil IM will induce menses of the endometrium if sufficiently primed with endogenous estrogen, and has proven to be safe in IVF and donor embryo cycles, where it routinely administered during the first 10 weeks of pregnancy.

Serum FSH, prolactin and estradiol tests may be rendered inaccurate for up to six weeks after the administration of OCs. Safer, more effective methods are available for diagnosis of pregnancy.

References for Section 2: Therapeutic Uses of OCs

1. Chiaffarino Francesca et al.: Oral contraceptive use and benign gynecologic conditions. Contraception 1998;57:11–18.
2. Royal College of General Practitioners. Oral contraceptives and health: An interim report from the oral contraception study of the Royal College of General Practitioners. New York: Pitman, 1974.
3. Vessey MP, Villard-MacKintosh L, Painter R: Epidemiology of endometriosis in women attending family planning clinics. Br Med J 1993;306:182–184.
4. Guillebaud J: Epidemiology of endometriosis. Letter to the editor. Br Med J 1993;306:931.
5. Cullberg G et al.: Effects of a low-dose desogestrel/EE combination on hirsutism, androgens, and sex hormone-binding globulin in women with polycystic ovary syndrome. Acta Obstet Gynecol Scand 1985;64(3):195–202.
6. Rojanasakul A et al.: Effects of combined desogestrel/EE treatment on lipid profiles in women with polycystic ovarian disease. Fertil Steril 1987;48(4):581–585.
7. Weiss NS et al.: Incidence of ovarian cancer in relation to use of oral contraceptives. Int J Cancer 1981;28:669–671.
8. Weiss NS, Sayvetz TA et al.: Incidence of endometrial cancer in relation to oral contraceptives. N Engl J Med 1980;302:551.

NOTES

SECTION 3: COMPOSITION AND EFFECTIVENESS

OC Composition

OCs are composed of synthetic estrogens and progestins (compounds with progestational properties) (1, 2).

Two synthetic estrogen and 12 synthetic progestin possibilities are available, although not all progestins are available in all countries. Estrogens and progestins vary in their biological activities (see Table 4).

The compositions and identifying characteristics of OCs available in the U.S. are shown in Table 5. OCs also contain inactive ingredients that act as fillers and preservatives. Rarely, women are allergic to the nonsteroidal contents (shown in footnotes of Table 4). When an allergic reaction occurs, it is most often due to lactose.

In combination OCs, the types and doses of estrogen and progestin remain constant during the 21 days that active tablets are taken, though the doses and ratios of estrogens and progestins vary from one preparation to another. Many combination OCs are also available in 28-day packages, which contain 21 active and seven inert or ferrous fumerate tablets.

In biphasic and triphasic OCs, the dose of the progestin or estrogen component changes during the cycle in an attempt to duplicate the pattern of the ovulatory menstrual cycle.

Progestin-only OCs contain no estrogen and are taken continuously. They are available in 28- and 42-day packages.

A new innovation is the extended use cycle in which active combination tablets are taken continuously for 84 days followed by 7 days of rest or inactive pills. This results in 9 additional weeks of OC use during a calendar year. In Table 6: Contraceptive Pill Activity, a correction is made in the activity of extended cycle regimen(s) by multiplying activity of a 21 day cycle employing the same ingredients by 1.23. At present only one extended cycle OC is available in the US but additional products are expected. Continuing OCs for 63 to 84 days without a break has been practiced by some physicians for a number of years, by having patients take 3 or 4 packs of 21-day OCs without a rest period between active pills.

Sequential preparations have been discontinued in the U.S. and Canada because of a possible increased risk of endometrial cancer. These regimens included 14 to 15 days of estrogen in doses above 50 mcg, followed by five to six days of estrogen and progestin.

Dose and Ratio of Estrogen and Progestin

Estrogen doses in OCs have ranged from 20 to 150 mcg. Since 1988, estrogen doses greater than 50 mcg have not been sold in the U.S. Progestin doses as high as 10 mg have been used in the past in combination OCs and from 0.05 to 1 mg in multiphasic OCs.

In the U.S., combination OCs now contain 0.1 to 1 mg of progestin. Progestin-only preparations may contain as little as 0.075 mg; multiphasic progestin preparations may contain as little as 0.05 mg on some days.

The ratio of estrogen-to-progestin in combination OCs ranges from 1:5 to 1:50, with the most commonly prescribed OCs having a ratio of 1:10 to 1:30. In the normal menstrual cycle, the ratio of active serum estrogen (estradiol plus estrone)-to-progesterone averages:
- 1:10 during the early follicular phase
- 1:5 during the pre-ovulatory phase
- 1:50 during the luteal phase.

OC Effectiveness

Contraceptive activity in OCs containing less than or equal to 50 mcg estrogen is primarily due to the progestin component. Progestin-only and combination OCs containing very low doses of progestin have slightly reduced effectiveness.

Contraceptive activity results from:
- Prevention of ovulation by suppression of hypothalamic and pituitary secretions (due to estrogenic and progestational actions)
- Alteration of cervical mucus to make it hostile to sperm (due to progestational and androgenic actions)

- Alteration of endometrial lining, preventing implantation (due to androgenic and progestational actions).

Pregnancy while taking OCs may be due to:
- Method failure (lack of OC efficacy)
- Patient failure (omission of OCs)
- Concurrent use of other drugs (see Section 6).

Women who smoke have an increased chance of becoming pregnant while using OCs. Women who are overweight have an increased risk of pregnancy when taking OCs (3, 4) (See Section 11).

It is especially important that patients be advised not to miss taking their OCs when low-dose formulations are used.

Most contraceptive failures are due to patient error in the first months of OC use. For this reason, many practitioners advise women to use concurrent backup contraception with the first month of OC use (see Section 8).

Contraceptive effectiveness is expressed as the Pearl Index. This indicates the number of pregnancies that occur for every 1,200 cycles, or 100 women per year of use.

There is no significant difference in combined failure rates between OCs containing 20 to 35 mcg of estrogen and those containing 50 mcg, according to manufacturer's data submitted to the FDA at the time of new drug applications. The combined failure rate is that due to all causes. Combined failure rates are:
- 0.79 for OCs with 20 mcg estrogen
- 0.13 to 1.3 for OCs with 30 to 35 mcg estrogen
- 0.08 to 0.88 for OCs with 50 mcg estrogen.

The differences in these reported failure rates are too small to justify using estrogen doses higher than 20 to 35 mcg even when highest contraceptive effectiveness is desired. However, the accidental omission of an OC pill may be more likely to result in pregnancy when low-dose combination or progestin-only OCs are used.

Family planning programs that have conducted independent studies show combination and multiphasic OC method failure rates of about 2.0 (5). This is higher than the rate reported by manufacturers. The combined pregnancy rate for OCs containing progestin only is 2.3 to 2.5.

Modern manufacturing practices are able to produce bioequivalent OCs with the same potency and effectiveness as the index brands. In the past, rare incidences of lack of potency occurred with index brands due to packaging. This can be a problem in tropical and subtropical zones unless OCs are enclosed in moisture-proof packaging and are stored at moderate temperatures. Current FDA guidelines recommend that OCs should remain stable when stored at temperatures between 15° and 30° C (59° and 86° F) at 60% humidity for 90 days. The FDA is considering revision of these guidelines. International guidelines specify that OCs should remain stable at 25° C (77° F) + 2%, at 60% + 5% relative humidity, for long-term stability, and at 40° C (105° F) + 2°, at 75% + 5% relative humidity, for short-term stability. Some bioequivalent OCs already meet international guidelines for stability.

References for Section 3: Composition and Effectiveness

1. Dickey RP: The pill: Physiology, pharmacology, and clinical use. In: Seminar in Family Planning, 1st ed. Isenman AW, Knox EG, Tyrer L (eds.) American College of Obstetrics and Gynecology, 1972. 2nd ed., 1974.

2. Dickey RP, Dorr CH II: Oral contraceptives: Selection of the proper pill. Obstet Gynecol 1969;33:273.

3. Talwar PP, Berger GS: Side effects of drugs: The relation of body weight to side effects associated with oral contraceptives. Br Med J 1977;1:1637–1638.

4. Holt VL, Cushing-Haugen KL, Daling JR. Body weight and risk of oral contraceptive failure. Obstet Gynecol 2002;99:820–7.

5. Sparrow MJ: Pregnancies in reliable pill takers. New Zealand Med J 1989;102:575–577.

SECTION 4: COMPARATIVE ACTIVITIES OF OCs

TYPES OF BIOLOGICAL ACTIVITY

In addition to contraceptive activity or efficacy (see Section 3), OCs have five major types of biological activities. These are:

- Estrogenic activity
- Progestational activity
- Androgenic activity
- Endometrial activity
- Effect on serum lipoproteins.

Table 4 lists the biological activities of individual contraceptive components (estrogens and progestins); Table 6 lists the biological activities of individual OCs.

The biological activity of an OC is a result of the combined activities of the estrogen and progestin components (1, 2, 3). Because of differences in the makeup of these components, each OC formulation has a different pattern of biological activity (4, 5). The results of the estrogenic, progestational, and androgenic activities may be seen in the side effects that occur when an excess or deficiency of one of the steroid components occurs (see Table 11) (6, 7) and in effects on serum lipids (see Table 7) (8, 9, 10, 11, 12, 13).

PROGESTIN STRUCTURE/ ACTIVITY RELATIONSHIPS

Most progestins used in the original OCs introduced in the early 1960s were structurally similar to androgens, except that they lacked a methyl (CH_3) group at the 19 position. The term 19-nor-progestin was used to describe these compounds, and they were named, as a group, the estrane progestins.

The first-generation 19-nor-progestins (norethin-drone [norethisterone]) contained only this change, plus the addition of an ethinyl group at the 17 position, which markedly

16

increases the activity of any steroids taken orally. Norethynodrel, the first 19-nor-progestins to be employed in an OC (Enovid®), had in common with estrogens a double-bond between the five and 10 positions (between the A and B rings) rather than between the four and five positions. As a result, norethynodrel, unlike norethindrone (norethisterone), had no androgenic activity and had more estrogenic activity than other 19-nor-progestins.

The second-generation of OC progestins were estrane compounds to which acetate groups were added at the 17 position (norethindrone acetate [norethisterone acetate]) or at both the 17 and three positions (ethynodiol diacetate or ethynodrel diacetate). Both of these additions increased overall progestational activity. Androgenic activity was increased by the acetate at the 17 position (norethindrone acetate) and decreased by an acetate at the three position (ethynodiol diacetate).

In the third-generation 19-nor-progestins, a methyl group was attached to the C-18 methyl group to create an ethyl group at C-13, creating the gonane group of progestins (dl-NG, LNG). These compounds had increased progestational potencies compared to estrane progestins and were also more androgenic. In addition, they completely lacked estrogenic activity (14).

In fourth-generation progestins, the 13-ethinyl gonane structure has been modified further by the addition of a methylene group at the 11 position (desogestrel), the addition of an acetate group at the 17 position, and the addition of a nitrogen at the three position (norgestimate) or the introduction of a double-bond between the 15 and 16 positions into ring D (gestodene). The 11-methylene group increases the binding to the progesterone receptor and reduces binding to the androgen receptor compared to LNG. The 15-to-16 double-bond increases binding only to the progesterone receptor, while binding to the androgen receptor is unchanged (15, 16, 17).

Pregnane progestins are structurally similar to progesterone. These include drospirenone and medroxyprogesterone acetate. Drospirenone is an analogue of spironolactone, an aldosterone antagonist with antimineralIcorticoid and antiandrogenic activities. Drospirenone counteracts the estrogen induced stimulation of the rennin-angiotensin system and blocks testosterone from binding to androgen receptors.

The activities of some progestins occur only after metabolism to a different compound (the active metabolite) in the liver and intestinal wall. Thus, estrane progestins are metabolized to norethindrone (norethisterone). For fourth-generation progestins, the changes to active metabolites are desogestrel to 3-keto desogestrel (Etonogestrel) and norgestimate to LNG.

Mestranol is metabolized to EE before combining with the estrogen receptor.

BIOLOGICAL ACTIVITY/ INDIVIDUAL OC ACTIVITY

The clinical actions of OCs are based primarily on the activities of the progestin and estrogen components and not on amount of drug. An OC's endometrial, estrogenic, progestational, and androgenic activities are dependent on the biological activities and the doses of individual estrogen and progestin components and by potentiating and antagonistic effects of one steroid component upon the other (1, 2, 3, 4, 5, 18, 19). The endometrial, estrogenic, progestational, and androgenic activity profiles of individual OCs are shown in Table 6.

Progestational, androgenic, and estrogenic activities of individual progestins are determined by animal and receptor assays (20, 21, 22, 23, 24, 25).

Endometrial activity is expressed in Table 6 as a percentage of patients who experience spotting, BTB, or early withdrawal bleeding (onset of menses before last active pill has been taken) during the third cycle of OC use. These are combined, since the distinctions among spotting, BTB, and early withdrawal bleeding are arbitrary from one manufacturer to another. The occurrence of spotting and/or BTB is always highest during the first cycle of OC use, decreases during the next two to three cycles, and changes little thereafter. Endometrial activity is related to estrogen dose and progestational and androgenic activities (3).

The effects of OCs on serum lipoproteins are shown in Table 7. The adverse lipid effects of OCs are related to the androgenic potential of the progestins and are mitigated by estrogen. OCs with higher ratios of estrogen-to-progestin or certain progestins, such as desogestrel or gestodene, have favorable effects of increasing serum HDL-cholesterol levels and decreasing LDL-cholesterol (13, 26, 27, 28, 29). Progestins and OCs with higher androgenic activities or lower estrogen-to-progestin ratios have unfavorable effects of lowering serum HDL-cholesterol, raising LDL-cholesterol, and increasing the ratio of total cholesterol divided by HDL-cholesterol.

The clinical significance of small decreases in LDL-cholesterol is unknown; however, it is generally believed that a 1% increase in LDL-cholesterol corresponds to a 2% increase in risk of cardiovascular disease (30).

References for Section 4: Comparative Activities of OCs

1. Chihal HJW, Dickey RP, Peppler R: Estrogen potency of oral contraceptive pills. Am J Obstet Gynecol 1975,121:75–83.

2. Dickey RP, Chihal HJW, Peppler R: Potency of three new low-estrogen pills. Am J Obstet Gynecol 1976;125:976–979.

3. Dickey RP, Stone SC: Progestational potency of oral contraceptives. Am J Obstet Gynecol 1976;47:106–111.

4. Dickey RP: Oral contraceptives: Basic considerations. In: Human Reproduction, Conception, and Contraception. 2nd ed. Hafez ESE (ed.) Hagerstown, PA: Harper and Row, 1978.

5. Dickey RP: The pill: Physiology, pharmacology, and clinical use. In: Seminar in Family Planning, 1st ed. Isenman AW, Knox EG, Tyrer L (eds.) American College of Obstetrics and Gynecology, 1972. 2nd ed., 1974.

6. Dickey RP: Diagnosis and management of patients with oral contraceptive side effects. J Cont Educ Obstet Gynecol 1978;20:19.

7. Dickey RP, Dorr CH II: Oral contraceptives: Selection of the proper pill. Obstet Gynecol 1969;33:273.

8. Godsland IF et al.: The effects of different formulations of oral contraceptive agents on lipid and carbohydrate metabolism. N Engl J Med 1990;323:1375–1381.

9. Knopp RH et al.: Oral contraceptive and postmenopausal estrogen effects on lipoprotein, triglyceride, and cholesterol in an adult female population: Relationships to estrogen and progestin potency. J Clin Endocrinol Metab 1981;53:1123.

10. Roy S et al.: The metabolic effects of a low-estrogen/low-progestogen oral contraceptive: Proceedings of a symposium. New York: Biomedical Information Corporation, 1981;24.

11. Speroff L, DeCherney A, et al.: Evaluation of a new generation of oral contraceptives. Obstet Gynecol 1993;81:1034–1047.

12. Wahl P et al.: Effect of estrogen/progestin potency on lipid/lipoprotein cholesterol. N Engl J Med 1983;308:862.

13. Wynn V, Nathyanthas R: The effects of progestins in combined oral contraceptives on serum lipids with special reference to high-density lipoproteins. Am J Obstet Gynecol 1982;142:766.

14. Phillips A et al.: Progestational and androgenic receptor binding affinities and in vitro activities of norgestimate and other progestins. Contraception 1990;41:399–410.

15. Kloosterboer HJ, Deckers GHJ: Desogestrel: A selective progestogen. Int Proc J 1989;1:26–30.

16. Kloosterboer HJ, Vonk-Noordegraaf CA, Turpijn EW: Selectivity in progesterone and androgen receptor binding of progestins used in oral contraceptives. Contraception 1988;38:325–32.

17. op ten Berg, M: Desogestrel: Using a selective progestogen in a combined oral contraceptive. Advances In Contraception 1991;7:241–250.

18. Gurpide E: Antiestrogenic actions of progesterone and progestins in women. In: Progesterone and Progestins. Bardin CW, Milgrom E, Mauvais-Jarvis P (eds.) New York: Raven Press, 1983;149–161.

19. Jung-Hoffmann C, Kuhl J: Interaction with the pharmacokinetics of EE and progestogens contained in oral contraceptives. Contraception 1989;40:299–312.

20. Bergink EV: Binding of contraceptive progestogens to receptor proteins in human myometrium and MCF-7 cells. Br J Fam Plann 1984;10:33.

21. Greenblatt RB: Progestational agents in clinical practice. Med Sci 1967;5:37–49.

22. Jones RC, Edgren RA: The effects of various steroids on vaginal histology in the rat. Fertil Steril 1973;24:284–291.

23. Phillips et al.: Comprehensive comparison of the potencies and activities of progestogens used in contraceptives. Contraception 1987;36:181.

24. Swyer GIM, Little V: Clinical assessment of orally active progestogens. Proc R Soc Med 1962;55:861–868.

25. Swyer GIM, Little V: Clinical assessment of relative potency of progestogens. J Repro Fertil 1968;5(suppl):63–68.

26. Beck P: Effect of progestins on glucose and lipid metabolism. Ann NY Acad Sci 1977;286:434–445.

27. Bradley D et al.: Serum high-density lipoprotein cholesterol in women using oral contraceptives, estrogens, and progestins. New Engl J Med 1978;299:17–20.

28. Wynn V et al.: Comparison of effects of different combined oral contraceptive formulations on carbohydrate and lipid metabolism. Lancet 1979;1:1045–1049.

29. Wynn V, Doar JWH, Mills GL: Some effects of oral contraceptives on serum lipid and lipoprotein levels. Lancet 1966;2:720–723.

30. Beller FK et al.: Effects of oral contraceptives on blood coagulation: A review. Obstet Gynecol Surv 1985;40(7):425–436.

SECTION 5: MANAGING SIDE EFFECTS

An important reason that women discontinue OC use is the experience of some associated side effects. A 1998 study found that the most common side effects that cause women to stop taking OCs while still needing contraception were (1):

- Bleeding irregularities—32%
- Nausea—19%
- Weight gain—14%
- Mood swings—14%
- Breast tenderness—11%
- Headache—11%.

Clinical Information

The steroid components of OCs produce effects in the body similar to those caused by the natural sex steroids produced in the ovaries. However, OC steroids differ from ovarian steroids in their:

- Pathways of entry into the main bloodstream:
    - OC steroids enter the hepatic circulation via the gastrointestinal (GI) tract and portal vein
    - Ovarian hormones enter the systemic circulation via ovarian veins and the inferior vena cava, bypassing the liver
- Blood level patterns:
    - OC steroids are administered as a single, large once-per-day dose
    - Ovarian hormones are continuously secreted in small amounts that vary throughout the menstrual cycle in levels and ratios of estrogen- to-progesterone
- Independence of pituitary regulation:
    - OC steroids are not under the control of the negative feedback from the pituitary
    - Ovarian steroids are under pituitary regulation
- Duration of action:
    - OC steroid action is prolonged due to modification of the structure
    - Ovarian steroids have a shorter duration of action

- Biological activities:
  - OC steroids may include androgenic and anti-estrogenic activities
  - Ovarian steroids do not include androgenic and anti-estrogenic activities
- Action at steroid receptors:
  - OC steroids may react differently than ovarian hormones.

Causes of Side Effects

Side effects occur when the hormone activity of an OC is either greater or less than the hormone effect of a woman's own ovarian steroids (2, 3).

Women taking OCs containing 50 mcg or less of estrogen usually have lower levels of the hormone acting on their reproductive tissues than they formerly received from their own ovarian steroids.

All women taking OCs have higher levels of sex steroids in the GI tract and liver, regardless of the OC dose, a situation that causes changes in many blood components manufactured in the liver (see Table 10).

Classification of Side Effects

Parallels to nearly all side effects of hormone excess from OC use may be found in the symptoms and physiological changes of pregnancy (3, 4). Parallels to the side effects of hormone deficiency can be found in the symptoms and changes of the pre- and post-menopausal periods. Table 11 contains a list of the most common side effects, classified according to their relation to an excess or a deficiency of hormone activity in the estrogen and/or progestin components.

Management

The first step in management of any symptom is to decide if the symptom indicates the presence or potential development of serious illness (see Table 12). If so, OCs must be discontinued immediately.

Some signs and symptoms may be potentially serious but do not necessitate immediate discontinuance of OCs. Women with such symptoms may continue taking OCs for a short time while they are being evaluated. These symptoms are also shown in Table 12.

The second step in the management of a side effect is to identify its probable cause. The center index of this text shows a grouping of side effects according to the body systems affected.

Side effects are addressed according to:
- Their probable cause
- The component of the OC most likely to be responsible
- Whether the side effect is due to an excess or a deficiency of OC component
- Suggested means of management.

The third step in the management of side effects is to make a decision about the probable clinical course of the side effect if OCs were to be continued. Some symptoms that occur in the first cycle of OC use (e.g., breakthrough bleeding (BTB) and side effects related to estrogen excess) will diminish or disappear spontaneously by the second or third cycle of use as the body becomes adjusted to the lower hormone level.

Women should be informed about possible side effects, and instructed to report their occurrence. Women need to know:
- Which side effects commonly occur during the first three cycles of OC use and may diminish or disappear spontaneously (see Table 11)
- Which side effects may be serious and require prompt medical attention (see Table 12)
- That their particular medical conditions or family histories make certain side effects more likely to occur.

If it has been determined that the side effect is OC-related, is not dangerous, and will not diminish or disappear spontaneously, the final step in the management of side effects is to switch a patient to an OC product that has a greater or lesser activity of the hormone that is causing the undesirable effect.

Table 6 lists OCs according to their four principal activities:

- Endometrial
- Progestational
- Estrogenic
- Androgenic.

A switch to an OC with equal or greater endometrial activity can be made at any time during the menstrual cycle. However, a switch to an OC with less endometrial activity should be made at the beginning of the next OC cycle in order to reduce the likelihood of BTB.

References for Section 5: Managing Side Effects

1. Rosenberg Michael J, Waugh Michael S: Oral contraceptive discontinuation: A prospective evaluation of frequency and reasons. Am J Obstet Gynecol 1998;179(3):577–582.

2. Dickey RP: Diagnosis and management of patients with oral contraceptive side effects. J Cont Educ Obstet Gynecol 1978;20:19.

3. Dickey RP, Dorr CH II: Oral contraceptives: Selection of the proper pill. Obstet Gynecol 1969;33:273.

4. Dickey RP: The pill: Physiology, pharmacology, and clinical use. In: Seminar in Family Planning, 1st ed. Isenman AW, Knox EG, Tyrer L (eds.) American College of Obstetrics and Gynecology, 1972. 2nd ed., 1974.

SECTION 6: DRUG INTERACTION

Clinical Information

Many patients take more than one drug simultaneously. Due to the length of time women take OCs, the possibility of concomitant therapy for coincidental disease is increased.

Drug interactions with OCs are of two types:
- Effects of other drugs on OC activities (see Table 14)
- Effects of OCs on other drugs (see Table 15).

6.

The interactions shown in Table 14:
- Reduce the efficacy of OCs
- Increase the side effects of OCs.

For patients well established on OCs, the unexpected occurrence of breakthrough bleeding (BTB) or spotting may be the first indication of drug interaction. In such a case, OCs may lose contraceptive effectiveness and pregnancy could result.

Antacids and isoniazid are no longer included in the list of drugs that interfere with OC action or absorption.

Mechanism of Interaction

OC steroids are weak inhibitors of hepatic microsomal drug oxidation (i.e., microsomal hydroxylating enzymes). As a result, the clearance of other drugs may be reduced, resulting in higher plasma concentrations (1).

OC steroids also enhance glucuronosyltransferase activity, thus enhancing hepatic conjugating capacity. This results in an increased clearance and, thus, lowering of plasma concentrations of drugs that are ordinarily eliminated by glucuronidation (2).

OC steroids may also influence the use of drugs to treat disease states by altering disease processes. For example, serum insulin levels and glucose levels are slightly elevated by OCs.

Many drugs are converted into water-soluble degradation products by enzymes. The rate of formation of these enzymes can be increased by different drugs:

- Barbiturates
- Anticonvulsant drugs
- Hypnotics
- The estrogen component of OCs.

One effect of enzyme induction is to accelerate the metabolism of the estrogen component of OCs.

Rifampin selectively reduces plasma levels of progestin (3, 4). Barbiturates reduce plasma levels of estrogen only. Antibiotics may interfere with intestinal intraluminal regeneration of OC steroids from their sulfate conjugates, thereby decreasing their availability during enterohepatic recycling.

A few drugs increase blood levels of OC steroids, principally estrogen, by inhibiting cytochrome P450 oxidation, among these are fluconazole (5), used for treatment of vaginal candidiasis, and ascorbic acid (6).

Management

A full drug history should be taken from all OC users. Patients should be warned of the possibility of drug interactions and of the loss of OC effectiveness if they take other drugs concurrently with OCs (4, 7, 8). They also should be instructed to inform other physicians and their pharmacists that they are taking OCs whenever other drugs are prescribed.

Additional contraceptive measures should be continued for one full cycle after discontinuing drugs that interfere with OC actions. Increasing OC dosages does not guarantee contraceptive efficacy and is the least desirable method of management.

There are some benzodiazepines (e.g., bromazepam and clotiazepam) and some corticosteroids (e.g., fluocortolone) whose activities are not increased by OC use. Valproic acid is one example of an anticonvulsant drug whose effectiveness is not decreased by OC use (9).

References for Section 6: Drug Interactions

1. Abernethy DR, Greenblatt DJ, Divoll M, Arendt RL: Impairment of diazepam clearance with low-dose oral contraceptive steroid therapy. Clin Pharmacol Ther 1984;35:360–366.

2. Legler UF: Lack of impairment of fluocortolone disposition in oral contraceptive users. Europ J Clin Pharm 1988;35:101–103.

3. Back DJ et al.: The effect of rifampicin on norethisterone pharmacokinetics. Eur J Clin Pharmacol 1971;15(3):193–197.

4. Dickinson B, Altman RD, Nielsen NH, Sterling ML. Drug interactions between oral contraceptives and antibiotics. Obstet Gynecol 2001;98:853–60.

5. Hilbert J, Messig M, Kuye O, Friedman H. Evaluation of interaction between fluconazole and an oral contraceptive in healthy women. Obstet Gynecol 2001;98:218–23.

6. Back DJ, Orme ML'E. Pharmacokinetic drug interactions with oral contraceptives. Clin Pharmacokinet 1990;18:472–84.

7. Sparrow MJ: Pill method failures. New Zealand Med J 1987;100:102–105.

8. Sparrow MJ: Pregnancies in reliable pill takers. New Zealand Med J 1989;102:575–577.

9. Crawford P, Chadwick D, Cleland P, Tjia J, Cowie A, et al.: The lack of effect of sodium valproate on the pharmacokinetics of oral contraceptive steroids. Contraception 1986;3:23–29.

NOTES

SECTION 7: TEENAGERS AND OCs

Louise Tyrer, M.D.
Former Vice President for Medical Affairs
Planned Parenthood Federation

Medical Aspects

Serious health risks from OC use are lower for women younger than age 20 than for other age groups. The estimated risk of death from OC use among teenagers is 1.3 per 100,000 users, while the risk of death in childbirth for this age group is 11.1 per 100,000 live births (1). Significant benefits from OC use include reductions in:

- Incidence of ovarian and endometrial cancers (continuing through later life) (2, 3)
- Pelvic inflammatory disease (PID)
- Follicular ovarian cysts
- Ectopic pregnancy
- Excessive menstrual bleeding
- Excessive cramps
- Endometriosis
- Acne vulgaris, including subsequent disfigurement.

Assessment

Health professionals evaluating teenagers for contraceptive needs should:

- Obtain family health profiles
- Obtain personal histories, including menstrual patterns and frequencies of intercourse
- Perform and assess physical examinations and indicated laboratory work
- Counsel about risks of pregnancy vs. various contraceptive options.

It is advisable that clinicians assure that onset of regular ovulation and menses has occurred prior to initiation of OCs for teenagers. However, adolescent girls with oligomenorrhea may have significantly higher androgen levels than those with normal cycles (4). OCs may relieve symptoms of excess androgen and irregular menses in these girls and may ameliorate the later development of polycystic ovarian syndrome (PCOS). Oligomenorrheic girls may temporarily experience increased fertility or revert to their original oligomenorrheic anovulatory states when they discontinue OC use. In the latter case, these patients may experience problems conceiving and require an infertility treatment latter in life.

Social Issues

Unintended teen pregnancy often results in the truncation of young women's education, thus limiting their opportunities to gain the skills needed to compete in society successfully (5). A teenage mother is more likely to be a single parent, to be divorced or separated, or to live in poverty, than are mothers of other age groups. Although six in 100 OC users younger than age 22 will become pregnant during their first year of OC use, the failure rate is four times higher for those using condoms and six to seven times higher for those using spermicides (6). For these reasons, the majority of sexually active teenagers seeking contraception choose OCs. However, most teens could benefit from simultaneous use of OCs and condoms, since condoms also provide some protection against sexually transmitted diseases (STDs).

Management

Compliance with OC regimens and intolerance of minor side effects, such as breakthrough bleeding, may be problems for this age group. Therefore, closer supervision, with prompt adjustment of OC dosage when necessary, is essential.

References for Section 7: Teenagers and OCs

1. Tietze C: New estimates of mortality associated with fertility control. Fam Plann Perspect 1977; 9(2):74–76.
2. Scotlenfeld D, Engle RL Jr: Decreased risk of endometrial cancer among oral contraceptive users. N Engl J Med 1980;303:1045.
3. Weiss NS et al.: Incidence of ovarian cancer in relation to use of oral contraceptives. Int J Cancer 1981;28:669–671.

4. Siegberg R et al.: Sex hormone profiles in oligomenorrheic adolescent girls and the effect of contraceptives. Fertil Steril 1984; 41(6):888–893.

5. Tyrer LB: Oral contraception for the adolescent. J Repro Med 1984;29(7suppl):551–559.

6. Schirm A et al.: Contraceptive failure in the U.S.: Importance of social, economic, and demographic factors. Fam Plann Perspect 1982;14:68.

NOTES

SECTION 8: STARTING OCs

Physical Examination and Medical History

A complete medical history and physical examination should be taken prior to the initiation or reinstitution of OCs and at least annually during OC use. These physical examinations should include special reference to blood pressure, breasts, thyroid, abdomen, liver, and pelvic organs, including cervical cytology and relevant laboratory tests.

Initial Examination Findings

The initial physical and laboratory examinations should result in normal findings. The following laboratory tests are recommended initially:

8.

- Cholesterol (for women ages 40 and older who have family histories of heart disease), including high-density lipoprotein (HDL) and low-density lipoprotein (LDL)
- Fasting insulin and blood sugar (for women who have family histories of diabetes)
- Leiden factor V (for patients who have personal or family histories of venous thromboembolism [VTE]).

Absolute Contraindications

Oral contraceptives should not be used by women who have the following conditions:

- Thrombophlebitis/thromboembolic disorders
- A history of deep vein thrombophlebitis or thromboembolic disorders
- Cerebral vascular or coronary artery disease
- Known or suspected carcinoma of the breast
- Known or suspected carcinoma of the endometrium or known or suspected estrogen- dependent neoplasia
- Undiagnosed abnormal genital bleeding
- Cholestatic jaundice of pregnancy or jaundice with prior pill use
- Hepatic adenomas, carcinomas, or benign liver tumors
- Known or suspected pregnancy

34

- Markedly impaired liver function
- Benign or malignant liver tumor that developed during previous use of OCs or other estrogen-containing products
- Type II hyperlipidemia (hypercholesterolemia)
- Leiden factor V mutation.

Relative Contraindications

OCs should be used with caution and patients should be monitored closely or OCs should not be used at all by women with the following conditions:

- Migraine or vascular headache
- Cardiac or renal dysfunction
- History of diabetes
- Gestational diabetes or impaired glucose tolerance
- Diastolic blood pressure of 90 mm Hg or greater or hypertension by any other criteria
- Psychic depression
- Varicose veins
- Ages 35 and older for smokers*
- Sickle-cell or sickle cell-hemoglobin C disease
- Cholestatic jaundice during pregnancy
- Worsening of any chronic condition during pregnancy
- Hepatitis or mononucleosis during past year
- First-order family histories of nonrheumatic cardiovascular disease (CVD) before age 50
- Use of drugs known to interact with OCs
- Ulcerative colitis.

*Some physicians consider smoking after age 35 as an absolute contraindication

Instructions about Early Side Effects

Some side effects that are common during the first through the third cycles of OC use disappear spontaneously thereafter. These side effects include breakthrough bleeding (BTB) and spotting (see Section 20) and symptoms associated with early pregnancy, especially nausea.

Patients should be encouraged to wait until the third cycle of OC use before seeking a change in or considering discontinuing OCs unless the side effect is one of those associated with serious disease.

Patients should be informed about symptoms of potentially serious side effects and warned to discontinue OCs and seek medical assistance at once if such symptoms occur (see Tables 11 & 12).

Onset of Effectiveness

The synthetic steroids in OCs are not completely eliminated from the body within 24 hours; therefore, their effect is cumulative, with a buildup over several days. Maximum effectiveness may not be reached until after seven days.

Ovulation may not be prevented if OCs are started after the fifth menstrual cycle day. Forty-eight to 72 hours may be required before contraceptive actions such as changes in the cervix, uterus, or endometrium are sufficient to prevent conception.

Starting Day

When first taken, OCs should be started on the first through the fifth menstrual cycle days.

Sunday Start: Some patient package inserts recommend starting OCs on Sunday as an aid to memory. If OCs are to be started on a Sunday, patients should take their first tablets on the first Sunday after their menstrual periods begin. If the period begins on a Sunday, patients should take their first tablets that day.

Quick Start: Some now recommend starting OCs at the time of the office or clinic visit irregardless of the cycle day as a method of increasing compliance and continuation. Starting OCs after the 7th cycle day may result in some patients being pregnant at the time OCs are started and or becoming pregnant if additional contraceptive methods are not used.

A backup method, such as condoms or contraceptive foam, should be used for the first seven days of the initial cycles if pills are started later than the fifth cycle day. Use of backup contraception for the first cycle is wise with all OCs and is necessary for progestin-only OCs.

After the first cycle, OCs should be restarted no later than seven days after the last active OC has been taken.

Forgotten or Missed Tablets

To help them remember to take their pills, patients should be instructed to take their OCs at the same time each day. Patients are most likely to forget or skip pills during the first cycles of use. It is important that patients know what to do if they forget to take one or more OCs.

Consecutive OCs Omitted	Time in Cycle	Instructions to Patients
1	Anytime	Take missed OC immediately and next OC at regular time
2	First two weeks	Take two OCs daily for next two days; then resume taking OCs on regular schedule. Use additional contraception for the remainder of the cycle
2	Third week	Take two OCs daily until all active pills are taken; restart OC cycle with one pill daily within seven days. Use additional contraception until OCs are restarted and for the first seven days of OC use
3 or more	Anytime	Stop OCs; restart OCs within seven days with one pill daily. Use additional contraception through the first seven days of the next pill cycle

Modified from Tyrer (1)

37

If menstruation does not occur at the regular time, a pregnancy test must be performed. If menstruation does occur, OCs should be restarted either five days after the onset of menstruation (as for the first cycle of OCs) or seven days after the last active tablet, whichever is earlier.

SPECIAL SITUATIONS

Recent Pregnancy

The risk of thromboembolism is increased for up to four weeks postpartum. Ovulation rarely occurs before the fourth week following a term pregnancy (2). If a woman is not nursing and is not using prolactin-suppressing drugs (such as bromocriptine [Parlodel®, Sandoz]), she may be started on combination or multiphasic OCs four weeks postpartum without waiting for her first menstrual cycle.

When prolactin-suppressing drugs are used, ovulation may occur before the fourth week postpartum and OCs should be started by the 14th postpartum day. Progestin-only pills may be started immediately postpartum.

Nursing

Steroid components of OCs may be found in the breast milk of nursing mothers (3). Combination OCs may inhibit lactation. For these reasons, many physicians recommend that nursing mothers not start OCs until their infants are weaned. OCs used during nursing should contain very low doses of estrogen and progestin so that milk production is not inhibited and the amount of drug in the breast milk is minimized. (See Section 10 for additional information).

Recent Abortion

Because of increased risks of thromboembolism and the possibility of ovulation during the first cycle following spontaneous or induced abortion, OCs should be started immediately or, at the latest, seven days following a first-trimester (five to 13 weeks) abortion. Following a mid-trimester abortion, OCs should be started at the same time as they would following a full-term pregnancy and other contraceptive methods should be used until seven days after OCs are started.

Irregular Menstrual Cycles

Women with amenorrhea or infrequent menstrual cycles (oligomenorrhea) may start OCs at any time if they are not pregnant and no other contraindications exist. Additional contraceptive methods should be used for the first cycle. Menses may be induced within seven to 14 days with progesterone in oil 100 mg IM.

Women with amenorrhea and oligomenorrhea should be advised of the possibility of worsening of these conditions after they stop using OCs. However, patients with anovulatory cycles should be encouraged to use OCs rather than other contraceptive methods to reduce their risks of developing endometrial and ovarian cancers.

Concurrent Drug Therapy

Contraceptive effectiveness may be lessened and BTB and spotting may occur when OCs are taken concurrently with other medications (see Table 14).

Women requiring medications listed in Table 14 should use additional contraception during all OC cycles or use a different contraceptive method.

References for Section 8: Starting OCs

1. Tyrer LB: Suggested patient instruction concerning missed pills. Memorandum, New York: Planned Parenthood Federation of America, August 3, 1976.
2. Phillips et al.: Comprehensive comparison of the potencies and activities of progestogens used in contraceptives. Contraception 1987;36:181.
3. Krattenmacher Rolf: Drospirenone: Pharmacology and pharmacokinetics of a unique progestogen. Contraception 2000;62:29–38.

SECTION 9: STOPPING OCs

GENERAL INFORMATION

A delay in the resumption of normal menstrual cycles or in conception may occur after OCs are discontinued.

It is recommended that women delay conception for one to three months after discontinuing OC use.

When OCs are discontinued before reproductive capacity has ended and contraception is still desired, other effective methods of birth control, such as IUDs or surgical sterilization, are recommended. Barrier methods, e.g., diaphragms, condoms, and spermicidal agents, are less effective.

REASONS FOR STOPPING OCS

Side Effects

OCs should be stopped immediately whenever potentially dangerous side effects occur (see Table 12). Other contraceptive means should be selected for these women, since the risks associated with pregnancy are usually greater than those associated with OC use.

If OCs are stopped prior to the tenth day of active pills, menstruation may not occur; if it does occur, it may be prolonged. OCs should be taken for at least 10 days if safe and feasible.

Missed Menses

Clinical Information

The possibility of pregnancy must be considered for women whose menses have not occurred after the first cycle of OCs or after 45 days from their last menstrual periods. OCs should be withheld until pregnancy has been ruled out.

Women can become pregnant even if they have adhered to their prescribed OC regimens.

Causal Factors

The most common cause for absence of menses while taking OCs is lack of endometrial stimulation due to low estrogenic activity (see Section 20). Absence of menses because of low estrogenic activity is often accompanied by breakthrough bleeding (BTB) or spotting during the days when OCs are taken.

Management

When no menses occurs, a pregnancy test should be performed before OCs are restarted. Absence of menses is not harmful and most often occurs in the first cycles of OC use, although it may also occur after OCs have been used for many months because of endometrial atrophy.

If lack of menses is due to low estrogenic activity, the endometrial thickness will usually be less than 5 mm on pelvic ultrasound. If the woman is not pregnant, she may continue on the same OC or be switched to an OC with greater endometrial activity (one with less BTB and spotting) (see Table 6).

Length of OC Use

The most recent studies have shown that the length of OC use is not a major factor in the development of serious side effects. There is no need to stop OCs because of length of use.

Age of OC User

OCs are as safe as other conventional contraceptive methods (which may fail and result in pregnancy) for women up to age 45 who do not smoke and for women up to age 35 who do.

In 1990, the FDA instructed manufacturers to revise OC labels to reflect the current scientific opinion that the benefits of OC use for healthy, nonsmokers older than age 40 may outweigh possible risks. To minimize risks, older women should be cautioned to take the lowest dose combination formulation that is effective.

SURGERY AND/OR HOSPITALIZATION

Combination and multiphasic OCs should be stopped prior to elective surgery requiring hospitalization or immobilization of an extremity because of a two- to sixfold increased risk of venous thromboembolism (VTE) (1). Although the exact length of time necessary to avoid this risk is not known, OCs should be discontinued for at least four weeks before surgery or prolonged immobilization, if feasible. Progestin-only OCs need not be discontinued.

Other methods of birth control should be substituted for OCs if continued contraception is needed during this period.

OCs may be resumed after the period of bed rest or immobilization has ended.

RESUMPTION OF MENSES AFTER OC USE

Patients may experience a delay in resumption of normal menstruation after discontinuing OCs (2). For women whose cycles were regular before OC use, the delay will be brief and the first menstrual period should occur by the fifth week after the last tablet is taken. Women who had irregular or infrequent menses (oligomenorrhea) before taking OCs may have a delay of three months or longer before resuming their previous menstrual patterns. However, some women with previous irregular menses will have one or more regular menstrual cycles before resuming their former patterns.

Failure of resumption of menses may be the result of pregnancy or menopause.

It is important for physicians to inform patients who discontinue OCs that the absence of menses does not necessarily indicate pregnancy and that they should not stop using other contraceptive methods until pregnancy is confirmed by appropriate tests.

High levels of LH in menopause may cause urine pregnancy tests to be false-positive.

References for Section 9: Stopping OCs

1. Jackson WE: Oral contraceptives and renal and retinal complications in young women with insulindependent diabetes meliitus. JAMA 1994;271:1099–1102.
2. Josimovich JB et al.: Heterogeneous distribution of serum prolactin values in apparently healthy young women and the effects of oral contraceptive medication. Fertil Steril 1987;47:785.

NOTES

SECTION 10: OC EFFECTS ON PREGNANCY AND NURSING

PREGNANCY DURING OC USE

Effects on the Fetus/Teratogenic Effects

Recent studies do not confirm earlier reports cited in OC package inserts (1, 2, 3, 4) that suggested an increased risk of teratogenic effects to the fetus if a woman inadvertently takes OCs during early pregnancy (31 references thereto were cited in the 9th edition). As a result, the warning that formerly appeared in OC package inserts has been revised to recognize this fact (5). However,

- If pregnancy is confirmed while OCs are being taken, OCs should be stopped immediately
- Pregnancy that occurs during OC use may be associated with an increased incidence of:
  - Spontaneous abortion
  - Ectopic pregnancy.

10.

Spontaneous Abortion

In one study, the incidence of spontaneous abortion reported among current OC users was 26% (3).

Ectopic Pregnancy

Ectopic pregnancy, as well as intrauterine pregnancy, may occur in contraceptive failures; one study reported a slight increase in ectopic pregnancies among OC users over nonusers (3). The ratio of ectopic-to-intrauterine pregnancies is higher in progestin-only OC failures than in nonusers because OCs are more effective in preventing intrauterine than ectopic pregnancies. A meta-analysis found a reduced incidence of ectopic pregnancy in OC users compared to controls (odds ratio [OR] = 0.19) and a slight increase in former OC users compared to controls (OR = 1.2) (6).

Management

Patients who miss two consecutive periods should be advised to discontinue their OC regimens until pregnancy has been ruled out. The administration of progestin-only or progestin/estrogen combinations to induce withdrawal bleeding should not be used as a test for pregnancy.

PREGNANCY AFTER OC USE

Delay in Conception After OC Use

There is an average two-month delay in conception after OCs are discontinued, however, some women will become pregnant without delay (7, 8). The percentage of women able to conceive within 24 months after discontinuing contraception is similar to that of other methods.

Spontaneous Abortion After OC Use

It has been recommended that patients allow one to three normal menstrual cycles to occur after they discontinue OCs before attempting pregnancy and that other contraceptive methods be used during this time. One reason not to attempt pregnancy immediately after stopping OCs is to allow time for the endometrium to recover from OC suppression. This usually occurs within one month. There is no evidence that the overall incidence of spontaneous abortion, when corrected for other factors, increases when patients become pregnant during the first cycles after discontinuing OCs. A study by the Royal College of General Practitioners (RCGP) failed to find any increase in abortions in women who stopped OCs to become pregnant.

Multiple Pregnancies

Multiple pregnancies have been reported to be increased after OC use is discontinued. This may be related to increased conception rates in patients with polycystic ovary syndrome (PCOS) during the first few cycles after OCs are stopped.

Effects of Prior OC Use on Offspring

Several large studies found no evidence for increased chromosomal abnormalities or congenital malformations in children of women who used OCs within one to three months prior to becoming pregnant (9, 10, 11). A 1986 study found an increased incidence of neural tube defect in children of women who used OCs prior to conception (11). The same study found significantly more weight gain during pregnancy in recent OC users. Long-term follow-up of children whose mothers used OCs prior to conception found no significant difference in children of nonusers in height, weight, development, and intelligence quotient.

In 1990, the FDA-package-insert was changed to read "extensive epidemiological studies have revealed no increased risk of birth defects in women who have used oral contraceptives prior to pregnancy" (5).

Prenatal vitamins with 0.8 to 1.0 mg folic acid should be started prior to conception (ideally three months prior) in all women planning pregnancy.

LACTATION

Clinical Information

Combination OCs reduce the quantity and quality of breast milk and reduce the duration of lactation. Progestin-only OCs have a lesser effect on production of breast milk. Injectable progestins either do not affect or may increase milk production (12, 13, 14).

OC estrogens and progestins are found in human breast milk when OCs are taken during lactation (15, 16). The possible effect of this on the newborn is unknown. It was previously estimated that an OC with 50 mcg ethinyl estradiol (EE) transfers 0.1 mcg EE per 600 ml of breast milk to the nursing infant and that the progestin transfer is 0.1% or less of the daily OC dose. It is now established that, in the case of Levonorgestrel (LNG), 10% of the agent present in maternal circulation gets into the breast milk (17). A time-dependent decrease in maternal serum and increase in breast milk levels of LNG has been observed (18). Once transmitted to breast milk, LNG becomes accumulated with the passage of time, resulting in higher levels in breast milk. For this reason, infants should be breastfed immediately after the mother ingests her OC rather than waiting until two to eight hours afterward, as was previously recommended.

Management

The World Health Organization (WHO) places no restrictions on the use of progestin-only methods after six weeks postpartum in lactating mothers. However, use of combination and triphasic OCs by lactating women may not be desirable because of the OCs adverse effects of breast milk quantity and quality and the possibility of effects on the newborn (19). Progestin-only OCs and injections have less or no effect on quantity or quality of breast milk but may affect the newborn (13). There is no evidence that OCs need to be started before 14 days postpartum in order to prevent conception.

OCs may be helpful in reducing breast engorgement once nursing has been discontinued.

References for Section 10: OC Effects on Pregnancy and Nursing

1. Bracken MB: Oral contraception and congenital malformations in offspring: A review and meta-analysis of the prospective studies. Obstet Gynecol 1990;76(2):552–557.
2. Linn S et al.: Lack of association between contraceptive usage and congenital malformations in offspring. Am J Obstet Gynecol 1983; 147(8)923–928.
3. Pardthaisong T, Gray RH: In utero exposure to steroid contraceptives and outcome of pregnancy. Am J Epidermiol 1991;134:795–803.
4. Polednak AP: Exogenous female sex hormones and birth defects. Pub Health Rev 1985;13(1–2):89–114.
5. Federal Drug Administration Drug Bulletin. April 1990;5.
6. Mol BWJ, Ankum WM, Bossuyt PMM, Van der Veen F: Contraception and the risk of ectopic pregnancy: A meta-analysis. Contraception 1995;52:337–341.
7. Pardthaisong T, Gray RH: The return of fertility following discontinuance of oral contraceptives in Thailand. Fertil Steril 1981; 35:532.
8. Vessey MP et al.: Fertility after stopping different methods of contraception. Br Med J 1978;1:265–267.

9. Harlap S et al.: Chromosomal abnormalities in the Kaiser-Permanente Birth Defects Study, with special reference to contraceptive use around the time of conception. Teratology 1985;31(3):381–387.

10. Harlap S, Shino PH, Ramcharan S: Congenital abnormalities in the offspring of women who used oral and other contraceptives around the time of conception. Int J Fertil 1985;30(2):39–47.

11. Magidor S et al.: Long-term follow-up of children whose mothers used oral contraceptives prior to conception. Contraception 1984;29(3):203–204.

12. Hull VJ: The effects of hormonal contraceptives on lactation: Current findings, methodological considerations, and future priorities. Stud Fam Plann 1981;12(4):134–155.

13. Jimenez J et al.: Long-term follow-up of children breastfed by mothers receiving depomedroxyprogesterone acetate. Contraception 1984;30(6):523–533.

14. Tankeyoon M et al.: Effects of hormonal contraceptives on milk volume and infant growth: WHO Special Programme of Research, Development, and Research Training in Human Reproduction. Contraception 1984;30(6): 505–522.

15. Laumas KR et al.: Radioactivity in the breastmilk of lactating women after oral administration of 3 H-norethynodrel. Am J Obstet Gynecol 1967;98:411–413.

16. Nisson S, Nygren KG: Transfer of contraceptive steroids to human milk. Res in Reprod 1979;11:1. 235. Norplant® package insert. Wyeth Laboratories, Inc., December 11, 1998.

17. Shikary ZK, Betrabet SS, Patel ZM, et al.: Transfer of LNG administered through different drug delivery systems from the maternal circulation into newborn infant's circulation. Contraception 1987; 35:477–486.

18. Toddywalla VS, Patel SB, Betrabet SS, Kulkarni RD, Saxena BN: Is time-interval between mini-pill ingestion and breastfeeding essential? Contraception 1995;51:192–205.

19. Madhavapeddi R, Ramachandran P: Side effects of oral contraceptive use in lactating women: Enlargement of breast in a breastfed child. Contraception 1985;32(5):437–443.

NOTES

SECTION 11: INITIAL
SELECTION OF OCs

(Also see Table 8)

CRITERIA FOR CHOICE OF OC

Factors to consider in choosing OCs are:
- Contraindications (see Section 8)
- Steroid dose
- Patient's personal/family health characteristics
- Patient's menstrual characteristics
- Patient's hormone sensitivity.

STEROID DOSE

Amount

The lowest dose and activity OC that is effective should be prescribed (1, 2). If feasible, OCs containing 35 mcg or less EE and the equivalent of 0.5 mg or less norethindrone should be used.

OCs with estrogen doses above 35 mcg may increase the incidence of thromboembolic disease.

There is no evidence that OCs with estrogen doses lower than 35 mcg reduce the risk of cardiovascular disease compared with OCs with estrogen doses of 35 mcg or more.

Progestins at doses as low as 1.0 mg norethindrone, 0.3 mg NG, or 0.15 mg LNG in combination pill regimens can cause significant changes in serum lipid and insulin levels, which may result in atherosclerotic vascular changes (see Table 7 and Section 26).

Selection of an OC with the appropriate dose and type of progestin significantly reduces the increased risks of cardiovascular disease.

Short- vs Long-Term Use

OCs containing more than 35 mcg estrogen and progestins with activities greater than 0.5 mg norethindrone may be necessary for short-term therapeutic use to decrease initial breakthrough bleeding (BTB) and spotting.

After one to three initial cycles, patients on higher-dose OCs should be switched to OCs containing 35 mcg or less estrogen and progestin with progestational and androgenic activities equal to 0.5 mg or less norethindrone if possible.

Multiphasic OCs in which estrogen and progestin doses are variable should contain total amounts of estrogen and progestin that do not exceed those of recommended combination OCs given for 21 days.

OCs that meet the presently recommended criteria for safe long-term use (e.g., that have less than 50 mcg estrogenic activity, low androgenic activity and no little or no adverse effects on serum lipids or clotting factors) are listed in Groups 1, 2, 5, 6, 7, 8, and 10 of Table 9.

Individual progestins may differ considerably in their progestational and androgenic activities (see Table 4). Doses of other progestins that result in activities equivalent to 0.5 mg norethindrone are:

- For progestational activity:
  - 0.05 mg gestodene
  - 0.06 mg desogestrel
  - 0.1 mg LNG (LNG)
  - 0.2 mg dl-NG
  - 0.25 mg Drosperone
  - 0.36 mg ethynodiol diacetate
  - 0.4 mg norgestimate
  - 0.43 mg norethindrone acetate
  - 1.0 mg drospirenone
- For androgenic activity:
  - 0.05 mg LNG (LNG)
  - 0.1 mg dl-NG
  - 0.15 mg desogestrel
  - 0.05 mg gestodene
  - 0.2 mg norgestimate
  - 0.3 mg norethindrone acetate
  - 0.8 mg ethynodiol diacetate.

Drospirenone has no androgenic activity.

PATIENT CHARACTERISTICS

Predisposing Factors to CVD

An increased risk of myocardial infarction (MI) and cerebrovascular accident (CVA) in OC users and nonusers is associated with the following factors:

- Type II hyperlipidemia (hypercholesterolemia)
- Diabetes mellitus
- Hypertension
- Obesity
- Smoking
- Leiden factor V mutation.

An increased risk of venous thromboembolism (VTE) is associated with:

- Obesity
- Varicose veins of the lower extremities
- Immobilization of a limb or of the entire body because of illness or surgery
- History of previous VTE.

(Also see Section 26)

Family History of CVD and Diabetes

A history of nonrheumatic CVD in first-order relatives before age 50 indicates a possible hereditary factor. OCs should not be used or should be used with caution by such women.

Because of the high incidence of maternal and fetal morbidity if they become pregnant, women who already have insulin-dependent diabetes should be allowed to take OCs or other steriod contraceptives when permanent contraception (sterilization of either partner) is unacceptable. There is no evidence that OC use increases renal or cardiovascular complications in women with insulin-dependent diabetes (3, 4). OCs with low, balanced doses of estrogen and low progestational activities should be chosen. If OCs are used, they should contain the lowest dose of progestin and estrogen compatible with normal menstrual cycles and patients should be monitored closely. (Also see Sections 26 & 27)

Age

The risks of both pregnancy and OC-related mortality increase progressively with age (see Table 2). Pregnancy-related mortality is six to seven times greater than OC-related mortality after age 30 in women who do not smoke. Mortality increases markedly after age 35 in OC users who do smoke. OC use is still safer than pregnancy until age 40 in women who smoke.

For women younger than age 18, there is no reason to refrain from prescribing OCs after regular menstrual cycles have been present for at least 12 months for treatment of the following conditions:
- Acne
- Contraception
- Regulation on menses
- Treatment of menstrual-related symptoms
- Other medical indications.

Height

Height growth usually ceases within one year of the first menses. Administration of sex steroids after menstruation starts does not appear to alter the final height attained.

Weight and OC Use

Underweight women are more likely to experience side effects of hormone excess.

However, underweight women have less BTB and spotting than over- and normal-weight women, and react most favorably to OCs with low estrogen doses and low progestational activities. Refer to Table 9, Groups 5, 7, 8 or any Triphasic.

Overweight women usually have more BTB and spotting during first cycles of OC use but, compared with normal to underweight women, have fewer minor side effects and less weight gain.

Overweight women may need OCs with higher endometrial activities initially. Two studies in 2002 (6) con-

53

firmed that women with higher body weight (> 70 kg/ had I 1/2 times the risk of contraceptive failure and this risk increased to 2 1/2 times if low dose OCs were used. Refer to Table 9, Groups 11, 12 and 13.

Ethnicity

Women of African and Middle Eastern origin have higher incidences of hypertension.

Women of Asian origin have increased sensitivies to estrogen but decreased sensitivities to progestins and progestin-related side effects (7).

Women of Northern European origin have higher incidence rates of venous thromboembolism (VTE).

Ethnic differences may be due to dietary or environmental differences and may change under different conditions.

MENSTRUAL CHARACTERISTICS
(Also see Table 8)

Clinical Information

The most frequent reason for patient dissatisfaction and discontinuance of OCs when contraception is still needed is menstrual irregularity (i.e., BTB and spotting) (8).

Bleeding irregularity is greatest during the first cycle of OC use and decreases thereafter until a plateau is reached in the third or fourth cycle (1). OCs that have high endometrial activities may be used during these early cycles to encourage continuation of use in new patients (2). However, in order to achieve the maximum possible menstrual control, there is no need to exceed limits of 50 mcg EE.

For initial cycles, side effects may be reduced if OCs are selected on the basis of a woman's menstrual pattern and history of sex steroid-related symptoms (see Table 8). However, choosing an OC in order to avoid one specific side effect may result in the occurrence of other side effects.

After the initial one to three cycles, all OC patients should be switched to formulations with sub-50 mcg estrogen doses and low or intermediate androgenic activities for continued long-term use (see Table 9, Groups 1 through 10).

Menstrual Types

OCs can be chosen on the basis of the following menstrual types (see Table 8):

- LIGHT FLOW AND MILD CRAMPS—Women with two to four days of light flow and mild or no cramps react favorably to OCs with low endometrial activities (see Table 9, Groups 3, 6, and 8)
- MODERATE FLOW AND AVERAGE CRAMPS— Women with four to six days of flow and average cramps may require OCs with slightly stronger endometrial activities during initial cycles (see Table 9, Groups 2, 4, 5, 7, 9, 10 and 11)
- HEAVY FLOW AND SEVERE CRAMPS—Women with six days or longer of flow and severe cramps require initial OCs with higher endometrial activities. In addition to requiring increased progestin doses or progestational activities, more estrogen (50 mcg) may be required to balance the increased progestational activity. High progestin doses (more than 1 mg norethindrone equivalent) should not be used by women with predispositions to hypertension (see Table 9, Group 13)
- IRREGULAR MENSES - Women with infrequent or irregular menses are often anovulatory.

Irregular Menses with Excess Androgen Effects

Irregular menses with excess androgen effects may be caused by polycystic ovaries or insulin resistance. Other causes that must be ruled out include:

- Ovarian tumors
- Adrenal tumors
- Adrenal hyperplasia.

Recommended OCs are those with high progestational and low androgenic activities (see Table 9, Groups 2, 6, 7, 8, and 10).

55

Irregular Menses without Androgen Effects

Irregular cycles or amenorrhea without androgen effects may be associated with:

- Exercise or dietary amenorrhea
- Pituitary tumor/hyperprolactemia
- Premenopause/menopause
- Diabetes
- Hypothyroidism.

Recommended OCs are those with low estrogenic and progestational activities (see Table 9, Groups 1, 5, and 8).

OCs should not be given to a woman with irregular cycles until a diagnosis has been established.

Women with infrequent or irregular cycles should be advised that they are likely to return to their former menstrual patterns when OCs are discontinued and that OCs may hide a progressive worsening of their conditions.

HORMONE SENSITIVITY

Clinical Information

Women may have experienced increased or decreased sensitivity to their own natural sex hormones. Evidence of this sensitivity may have occurred during periods of physiological hormone excess, such as pregnancy, or at the time of low hormone levels preceding or during menses (1, 2).

Estrogen-Sensitive Women

Symptoms of excessive sensitivity to estrogen are:

- Unusually severe nausea or edema during pregnancy or at menstrual midcycle
- Enlarged uterus
- Uterine fibroids
- Cervical hypertrophy
- Large or painful breasts
- Fibrocystic disease of the breast
- Heavy menstruation
- Severe cramps during menstruation.

Low estrogenic activity OCs should be chosen initially for these women (see Table 9, Groups 1, or any 20 mcg EE OC).

Progesterone-Sensitive Women

Signs and symptoms of progesterone sensitivity are:
- Premenstrual symptoms, including:
  - Edema
  - Abdominal bloating
  - Headache
  - Depression
- Pregnancy, symptoms such as:
  - Excessive appetite
  - Excessive weight gain
  - Excessive tiredness
  - Hypertension
  - Varicose veins.

Low progestational activity OCs should be chosen initially for these women (see Table 9, Groups 1, 8, and 10 (antimineralocorticoid activity), or any Tri-Phasic.

Estrogen-Deficient Women

Symptoms of estrogen insufficiency include:
- Scant menses
- Small uterus
- Small breasts
- Midcycle spotting.

Women with these symptoms or findings should not be given OCs with high estrogen contents initially, as has been occasionally suggested. Instead they should be started on 20 or 25 mcg EE combination OCs and the dose should be increased only if required (see Table 5). A lack of estrogenic effects may result from the physiological down-regulation of estrogen production; attempts to override this with excessive estrogen doses may result in side effects.

Progesterone-Deficient Women

Women with progesterone deficiency have symptoms similar to those of women with anovulatory cycles and corpus luteum insufficiency, including:

- Prolonged menses
- Heavy menses
- Severe cramping
- Premenstrual BTB or spotting
- Premenstrual symptoms.

Similar symptoms may occur due to endometriosis and adenomyosis. These women may require OCs with increased progestational and/or androgenic activities (see Table 9, Groups 2, 3, and 10).

Androgen-Sensitive Women

Women with excessive androgen effects may have:

- Oily skin
- Acne
- Male pattern hair growth.

Causes of excessive androgen effects, other than neoplasia and adrenal causes, require different treatment regimens:

- For women with high androgen and normal or high estrogen levels (polycystic or Stein-Leventhal ovaries), high-progestin/low-androgen combination OCs are recommended for suppression of ovarian androgen (see Table 9, Groups 2, 6, 7, 8, and 10)
- For women with normal androgen levels and low estrogen levels, because excess androgen symptoms are often due to low levels of sex hormone binding globulin (SSBG), OCs containing 30 mcg estrogen with low androgenic activity are recommended. (see Tables 5 and 6).

References for Section 11: Initial Selection of OCs

1. Dickey RP: Oral contraceptives: Basic considerations. In: Human Reproduction, Conception, and Contraception. 2nd ed. Hafez ESE (ed.) Hagerstown, PA: Harper and Row, 1978.

2. Dickey RP, Chihal HJW, Peppler R: Potency of three new low-estrogen pills. Am J Obstet Gynecol 1976;125:976–979.

3. Inman WHW et al.: Thromboembolic disease and the steroidal content of oral contraceptives: A report to the Committee on Safety of Drugs. Br Med J 1970;2:203–209.

4. Palatsi R, Hirvensalo E, Liukko P, et al.: Serum total and unbound testosterone and sex hormone binding globulin (SHBG) in female acne patients treated with two different oral contraceptives. Acta Derm Venereol (Stockh) 1984;64(6):517–523.

5. Talwar PP, Berger GS: Side effects of drugs: The relation of body weight to side effects associated with oral contraceptives. Br Med J 1977;1:1637–1638.

6. Holt VL, Cushing-Haugen KL, Daling JR. Body weight and risk of oral contraceptive failure. Obstet Gynecol 2002;99:820–7.

7. Walnut Creek Contraceptive Drug Study. Results of the Walnut Creek Contraceptive Drug Study. J Repro Med 1980;25(suppl):346.

8. Rhodes JM et al.: Colonic Crohn's disease and use of oral contraception. Br Med J (Clin Res) 1984;288(6417):595–596.

SECTION 12: EMERGENCY CONTRACEPTION

General Information

Awareness and use of emergency contraceptives (EC) has increased in the past two years and, when over-the-counter sales are approved, will increase even more. With increased use have come greater understanding of the parameters for use and side effects.

Time limit for initiating contraception

Initially it was believed that to be effective EC must be initiated within 72 hours of unprotected intercourse. This is still true for maximum effectiveness when hormonal contraceptive methods are used but is not true for mifepristone (MF) or IUD insertion. OC regimens can prevent pregnancy with a time related decrease in effectiveness as late as 5 days after unprotected intercourse. In two studies evaluating the Yuzpe regimen, effectiveness was 87 to 90% in preventing pregnancy when OCs were started within 72 hours compared to 72 to 87% when OCs were started 72 to 120 hours after intercourse (1, 2). A larger study that compared the Yuzpe regimen to 100 mg MF as a single dose—both initiated within 72 hours—concluded that the Yuzpe regimen was 56% effective in preventing pregnancy compared to 92% effectiveness of MF (3). An increasing coitus-to-treatment interval was associated with contraceptive failure in the Yuzpe group whereas no association was seen with MF. The Yuzpe regimen also had significantly fewer side effects than MF. A much larger study comprising >6000 women treated with 10 mg MF found a sharp decline in effectiveness when treatment was administered during the fifth day but this may have been because of the lower dose of MF (4). In the same study, 10 mg MF was 83% effective in preventing pregnancy. The risk of pregnancy was 28 times higher when women had additional acts of unprotected intercourse between the day of drug administration and menses, but an insignificant increase in risk if they had protected intercourse. The same

12.

authors found that pregnancy rates were not significantly higher when 5, 10, 25, or 50 mg of MF was administered compared to 100 mg of MF in a meta-analysis of >10,000 Chinese patients (5). The effectiveness of MF doses smaller than 100 mg in Western women has not been established. At present MF is not available for EC in the United States.

Emergency Contraceptive Drugs Available in the United States

The effectiveness of OC hormones for EC was established by the seminal paper of Yuzpe and colleagues published in 1977 (6). Prior to 1977, hormonal contraception was widely used by knowledgeable physicians but consisted of administration of high doses of conjugated estrogen IV or orally with the expected side effects (7, 8, 9). The Yuzpe regimen comprises NG 0.5 mg and EE 0.05 mcg (Ovral, Ogestrel)—two pills initially and two pills repeated in 12 hours (6). For 30 years this was standard treatment when EC was needed. Various other OCs could be substituted for Ovral (see the list, below) but these were always combination drugs given in two doses 12 hours apart.

Two recent discoveries have changed this. The first was that LNG, the active isomer of NG, could be used alone without estrogen for EC if the dose was high enough. The 0.75 mg dose of LNG in Plan B® represents 1.5 times the progestational and androgenic activity contained in one tablet of Ovral (see Table 5) or ten times the progestational and androgenic activity contained in one tablet of Ovrette 0.075 mg NG progestin OC. Despite the 50% higher progestational and androgenic activity, side effects, nausea and vomiting are significantly less common with LNG compared with NG/EE as are other symptoms estrogen related symptoms (headache, dizziness, fatigue, low abdominal cramping, and breast tenderness), and pregnancy rates are lower with LNG compared to NG/EE (1.17% vs. 3.2%) (10).

The second discovery was that LNG was even more effective if the entire 1.5 mg dose contained in two tablets was taken at one time (11). In this study of 1118 women, the estimated effectiveness was 87% for 0.75 mg LNG taken in two doses 12 hours apart, compared to 93% for 1.5 LNG in a single dose. The incidence of side effects headache, breast tenderness and heavy menses was higher in the high dose group, but the better compliance in clinical practice and higher rate of effectiveness were considered to offset this. This study also found that pregnancy rates increased with delay in starting treatment and if further acts of unprotected intercourse took place after treatment.

NG and LNG containing OCs that can be used for EC are shown in the following list. OCs containing other progestins are not recommended except when no NG or LNG pills are available. The reason is that the other OCs have not been extensively tested, and the higher androgen potency of NG and LNG may contribute to their effectiveness. A single study in which 1672 women were randomized to receive the standard Yuzpe regimen, norethindrone 2 mg + EE 100 mcg, or only the first two tablet dose of the Yuzpe regimen, the respective pregnancy rates were 2.0%, 2.7%, and 2.9% (12). Copper-wrapped IUDs can also prevent pregnancy, with 98% effectiveness in parous women and 92% effectiveness in nulliparous women, when used as late as five days after ovulation (13, 14).

OC and Other Pills Suitable for Emergency Contraception

OC formulas approved by the FDA for emergency contraception:
- Preven™—NG 0.5 mg/EE 0.05 mcg; two pills initially and two pills repeated in 12 hours.
- Plan B™—LNG 0.75 mg; one pill initially and one pill repeated 12 hours later.
  Alternative dosing for Plan B®; Two pills initially, no repeat (11).

Other recommended OCs equivalent to those approved by the FDA:
- In place of Preven™:
  - Ogestrel®, Ovral® 21 (NG 0.5 mg/EE 0.05 mcg); two pills initially and two pills repeated in 12 hours (15, 16)

- Levora®, Levlen®, LoOvral®, Low-Ogestrel®, Nordette® (NG 0.3 mg or LNG 0.15 mg/EE 0.03 mcg); four pills initially and four pills repeated in 12 hours
- Alesse®, Levlite® (LNG 0.1 mg/EE 20 mcg); five pills initially and five pills in 12 hours
- In place of Plan B™:
  - Ovrette® (NG 0.075 mg); 20 pills initially and 20 pills repeated in 12 hours

For additional information about Plan B® call *800–330–1271*.

Clinical Information

To be effective, postcoital contraceptive agents must be administered as soon as possible after unprotected coital exposure. When administered within 72 hours of intercourse, recognizable pregnancy occurs only 1.17% (LNG 0.75 mg) to 3.2% (NG-LNG 0.5 mg/EE 0.05mcg) of the time compared with an expected rate of 6.6%. Initiation of regimens within 24 hours of intercourse increases the chance that pregnancy will be prevented (17). Use of steroids for emergency contraception is not intended for repeated use. Women should be counseled to use OCs or other contraceptive methods regularly. There is one report of ectopic pregnancy after use of emergency contraception (18).

Side Effects

Delay in expected menses may occur. For patients taking either NG/EE or LNG, menses was delayed three to seven days in 15% and more than seven days in 13% of patients. Menses was early in 15% of patients (17). Early onset of menses and spotting following the use of EC is common. In an analysis of return of menses and bleeding rates in 1949 EC patients who received the Yuzpe regimen, Norethindrone + EE, or a single dose of two Ovral tablets described above (12), menses was more than 3 days early in 64% who were treated before the 12 day compared to 48% treated day 12–14, and

28% treated after day 14 (19). Spotting occurred in 10% of patients, and was unrelated to whether or not the treatment failed and patients became pregnant.

Patients who become pregnant after treatment with Mifepristone™ may be at increased risk of their offspring developing birth defects. Pregnancy after Mifepristone™ use has been associated with sirenomelia, or the mermaid syndrome in which the legs are fused (20).

References for Section 12: Emergency Contraception

1. Rodrigues I, Grou F, Joly J. Effectiveness of emergency contraceptive pills between 72 and 120 hours after unprotected intercourse. Am J Obstet Gynecol 2001;184:531–7.
2. Ellertson C, Evans M, Ferden S, Leadbetter C, Spears A, Johnston K, Trussell J. Extending the time limit for starting the Yuzpe regimen of emergency contraception to 120 hours. Obstet Gynecol 2003;101:1168–71.
3. Ashok PW, Stalder C, Wagaarachchi PT, Flett GM, Melvin L, Templeton A. A randomized study comparing a low dose of mifepristone and the Yuzpe regimen for emergency contraception. BJOG 2002;109:553–60.
4. Piaggio G, von Hertzen H, Heng Z, Bilian X, Cheng L. Combined estimates of effectiveness of mifepristone 10 mg in emergency contraception. Contraception 2003;68:439–46.
5. Piaggio G, von Hertzen H, Heng Z, Bilian X, Cheng L. Meta-analysis of randomized trials comparing different doses of mifepristone in emergency contraception. Contraception 2003;68:447–52.
6. Yuzpe AA, Percival-Smith R, Rademaker AW: A multicenter clinical investigation employing EE combined with dl-NG as a post-coital contraceptive agent. Fertil Steril 1982;37:508.
7. Cook CL et al.: Pregnancy prophylaxis: Parenteral postcoital estrogen. Obstet Gynecol 1986;67:331.
8. Morris JM, Van Wagenen G: Interception: The use of postovulatory estrogens to prevent implantation. Am J Obstet Gynecol 1973;115:101–106.
9. Van Santen MR, Haspels AA: A comparison of high-dose estrogens vs low-dose EE and NG combination in postcoital interception: A study in 493 women. Fertil Steril 1985;43(2):206–213.
10. Hjelt K et al.: Oral contraceptives and the cobalamin (vitamin B12) metabolism. Acta Obstet Gynecol Scand 1985;64(1):59–63.

11. Arowojolu AO, Okewole IA, Adekunle AO. Comparative evaluation of the effectiveness and safety of two regimens of levonorgestrel for emergency contraception in Nigerians. Contraception 2002;66:269–73.

12. Ellerston C, Webb A, Blanchard K, Bigrigg A, Haskell S, Shochet T, Trussell.Modifying the Yuzpe regimen of emergency contraception: a multicenter Randomized controlled trial. Obstet Gynecol 2003;101:1160–7.

13. Liyimg Z, Bilian X, Emergency contraception with a multiload Cu-375 SL IUD: a multicenter trial. Contraception 2001; 64:107–12.

14. Glasier A: Emergency postcoital contraception. New Engl J Med 1997;337:1058–1064.

15. Wynn V et al.: Effects of oral contraceptives on carbohydrate metabolism. J Reprod Med 1986;31(9 Suppl):892–897.

16. Wynn V, Doar JWH, Mills GL: Some effects of oral contraceptives on serum lipid and lipoprotein levels. Lancet 1966;2:720–723.

17. Ho PC, Kwan MSW: A prospective randomized comparison of LNG with Yuzpe regimen in postcoital contraception. Human Repro 1993;(8)3:389–392.

18. Kubba AAC, Guillebud J: Case of ectopic pregnancy after postcoital contraception with ethinyl oestradiol-LNG. Br Med J 1983;287:1343. 230 231

19. Webb A, Shochet T, Bigrigg A, Loftus-Granberg B, Tyrer A, Gallagher J, Hesketh C. Effect of emergency contraception on bleeding patterns. Contraception 2004;69:133–5.

20. Potts JC, Papernik E: Mifepristone teratogenicity. Lancet 1991;338:1332–1333.

SECTION 13: INJECTED CONTRACEPTIVES

Depo-Provera® Contraceptive Injections
(150 mg medroxyprogesterone acetate)

Status

The Depo-Provera® 150 mg IM injections at three-month intervals for contraception has been tested extensively in the U.S. since the 1960s and are used in more than 80 countries.

Pharmacology

MPA consists of a substituted C-21 molecule that is without androgenic or estrogenic effects. Inactive ingredients include polyethylene glycol, polysorbate, nace, methylparaben, and propylparben.

The androgenic side effects occasionally reported may be the result of decreased sex steroid-binding globulin.

Depo-MPA is a crystalline suspension that is insoluble in water and lipids. After injection, crystalline deposits form in tissue and are reabsorbed slowly. Peak levels of MPA reach 7 µg/ml three weeks after a 150 mg injection and 2 µg/ml ten days after the 25 mg injection. The area of MPA under the curve is 25% higher when injections are given in the arm than when they are given in the thigh or buttocks; however, their respective peak levels are not statistically different (1). MPA may be undetectable after four months but has been measured in serum as late as eight months after injection. MPA serum levels were not found to vary according to weight, body mass index or ethnicity in a study conducted in Black African, Indian, and White women in South Africa (2).

Onset of Action

MPA 150 mg every three months is 99% effective in suppressing ovulation if initially given before the eighth cycle day (3, 4). Changes in cervical mucus, a secondary mechanism of contraception, are not complete until the fourth to seventh cycle day (5, 6). After the first injection

13.

MPA 150 mg should be given every 12 weeks without regard to menstrual day.

Clinical Information

MPA 150 mg IM every three months has a failure rate of 0.25 to 0.3 per 100 women per year.

Side Effects

Side effects specific to MPA 150 mg are related to progestin excess and estrogen deficiency (see Table 11).

Up to 50% of women using MPA 150 mg experience breakthrough bleeding or spotting during their early cycles of use. By month 12, amenorrhea is reported by 55% of women; and by month 24, amenorrhea is reported by 68% of women using MPA (7). Galactorrhea may occur as a result of MPA use (8).

Bleeding is likely to be increased at the time of surgery if a hysterectomy is performed within six weeks of patients receiving MPA (author's experience).

Other side effects that occur significantly more often with MPA than with other hormonal contraception are:

- Decrease of bone density

  Use of MPA may be associated with bone loss. The rate of bone loss is greater in the early years of use, then subsequently approaches the normal rate in the time of age-related falls. Two years of contraception with MPA in adolescent girls was associated with an average 6.8% reduction in bone-mineral density compared to controls (Ob.Gyn. News, August 1, 2003). Women who used MPA through to menopause were found to have attenuated rates of bone loss from the lumbar spine and femoral neck, presumably because they had already lost the estrogen-sensitive component of bone (9).

- Weight gain

  Women who complete one year of MPA 150 mg gain an average of 5.4 lbs., which increases to 8.1 lbs. after two years and 13.8 lbs. after three years (1).

Laboratory Changes

MPA causes a 25-% decrease in triglyceride and HDL- and total cholesterol levels and causes a mild deterioration in glucose tolerance associated with an increased insulin response (10). Contrary to FDA labeling information, it has no effect on liver function.

Drug Interactions

Aminoglutethimide administered concomitantly with MPA may significantly depress serum concentrations (11).

Depression

Use of MPA does not increase or intensify episodes of depression (12).

Cardiovascular Risk

There is little or no increased risk of acute myocardial infarction, stroke, or venous thrombo-embolism in women who use 150 mg MPA (13).

Cancer Risk
Breast Cancer

Approval of Depo-Provera® IM as a contraceptive was postponed for more than two decades because of concerns about breast cancer. However, the risk appears to be small for long-term use and is balanced by a reduced risk of endometrial cancer. In 1996, the physician package insert for MPA contraceptive injections was changed to indicate the extent of breast cancer risk (1). The relative risk of breast cancer for women of all ages who had initiated use of MPA during the previous five years was 2.0 (95%, confidence interval [CI] 1.5 to 2.8) (14).

An increased relative risk (RR) of 2.19 of breast cancer has been associated with use of Depo-Provera® in women whose first exposure to the drug was within the previous four years, and were younger than age 35. This represents an additional 31.8 cases of breast cancer per 100,000 women ages 30 to 34 (95%). However, the overall relative risk for ever-users of Depo-Provera® was only 1.2 (15).

68

Use before age 25 was associated with a RR of 1.32, which increased with years of total use from 1.02 for less than one year to 2.41 for more than three years (15). The RR after age 25 was highest (1.39 to 1.42) during the first three years of use, and fell to 0.78 after three years. For all ages, the risk of a newly diagnosed breast cancer was less than 1.0 eight years after first use, regardless of continuation of use.

Cervical Cancer
A statistically insignificant increase in RR of invasive squamous cell cervical cancer has been associated with use of Depo-Provera® in women who were first exposed before the age of 35 (RR 1.22 to 1.28) (95% C.I. 0.93 1.70) (1, 16). The overall relative rate of invasive squamous cell cervical cancer in women who ever-used Depo-Provera was estimated to be 1.11 (95% C.I. 0.96 to 1.29). No trends in risk with duration of use or time since initial or most recent exposure were observed.

Endometrial Cancer
The risk of endometrial cancer may be reduced by use of MPA (17).

Ovarian Cancer and Liver Cancer
MPA is not associated with an increased risk of ovarian or liver cancer (18, 19).

Other Side Effects
There have been a few reported cases of convulsions in patients who were treated with MPA contraceptive injections (1). Fluid retention and breast tenderness may occur with MPA 150 mg.

Return of Fertility
Amenorrhea may continue for an extended time after MPA 150 mg IM. The average time to return to ovulation is five to eight months, and the average time to pregnancy is 10 months, with a range from four to three months. There have

been four anecdotal reports of permanent anovulation in new drug studies. Anovulation of longer than six months may be successfully treated with human menopausal gonadotropin (author's experience).

Effect on Fetus if Accidental Pregnancy Occurs

Infants from accidental pregnancies that occur one to two months after injection of MPA contraceptive injection may be at an increased risk of low birth weight, which in turn is associated with an increased risk of neonatal death. The attributable risk is low because such pregnancies are uncommon (20, 21).

A significant increase in incidence of polysyndactyly and chromosomal anomalies was observed among infants of MPA users, the former being most pronounced in women younger than age 30. The unrelated nature of these defects, the lack of confirmation from other studies, and the chance effects due to multiple statistical comparisons make a causal association unlikely (22).

Children exposed to MPA in while breastfeeding showed no evidence of any adverse effects on their health, including their physical, intellectual, sexual, and social development (23).

The risk of hypospadias (five to eight per 1000 male births in the general population) may be approximately doubled with exposure to progestational drugs.

Pregnancy and Lactation

Because progestational drugs may induce mild virilization of the external genitalia of the female fetus and because of the increased association of hypospadias in the male fetus, it is important that the first injection be given only during the first five days after the onset of a normal menstrual period in non-postpartum women and by the fifth day postpartum in non-nursing mothers.

Detectable amounts of the drug have been identified in the breast milk of mothers receiving MPA. No adverse effects have been noted for nursing mothers treated with

MPA contraceptive injection in breast milk composition, quality, and amount. Additionally, no adverse effects have been noted developmentally and behaviorally through puberty for infants exposed to MPA via breast milk (1). The patient information insert for Depo-Provera® for contraception warns that postpartum patients who are nursing should wait at least six weeks before starting MPA (1).

Persistent galactorrhea for more than six months after stopping nursing occurred in 64% of MPA users.

Management and Dose

Use of MPA 150 mg IM is indicated for conditions in which estrogen-containing OCs are contraindicated, when compliance is a problem, and for women older than 35 who smoke. The possibility of an extended interval until return to fertility must be understood and accepted by the patient.

The usual dose of MPA is 150 mg IM every three months. MPA is also effective at a dose of 400 mg IM every six months.

The addition of supplemental estrogen, in either IM or oral forms, for control of irregular menstruation and amenorrhea is not recommended.

MPA should not be re-administered if thrombolic disorders (i.e., thrombophlebitis, pulmonary embolism, cerebrovascular disorders, and retinal thrombosis) occur or are suspected.

MPA should not be readministered pending examination if there is a sudden onset of proptosis, diplopia, or migraine. Conditions that might be influenced by fluid retention, such as epilepsy, asthma, and cardiac or renal dysfunction, require careful observation.

Women who have histories of psychic depression should be carefully observed, and MPA should not be readministered if depression occurs.

Due to potential harm to the fetus, women who develop amenorrhea should have a urine pregnancy test before their next tri-monthly injection.

Lunelle™ Monthly Contraceptive Injections
(Recalled October 2002)
(25 mg medroxyprogesterone acetate with
5 mg estradiol cypionate)

Lunelle™, a once-per-month injection of 25 mg me-droxyprogesterone acetate (MPA) with 5 mg estradiol cypi-onate (EC), was FDA approved for U.S. use in 2000 and is sold in other countries under the name Cyclofem™ (4, 6). Lunelle™ prefilled syringes, which was the form in which most Lunell™ was supplied, were recalled in October 2002 because some lots were found to lack full potency indicating the potential of contraceptive failure. Lunelle™ was initially sold in the form of single dose vials which were not affected by the recall. At the time of recall approximately 100,000 women were using Lunelle™ in the US. Because of the lack of sufficient vials of Lunelle™ to replace the subpotency prefilled syringes all sales of Lunelle™ were suspended. No cases of pregnancy due to failure of the lots in question were reported (Ob. Gyn. News November 15, 2002). The manu-facturer had not reintroduced Lunelle™ for sale in the US as of May 1, 2004.

Lunelle™ had to be initially administered by the fifth cycle day, compared to the eighth day for Depo-Provera®. After the first cycle, Lunelle™ injections should be adminis-tered every 28 to 30 days without regard to the onset of menses, which may start earlier or be absent (1). MPA 25 mg with EC 5 mg every month had a failure rate of 0.06 per 100 women per year (24).

Side effects of Lunelle™ were similar to those for estrogen-containing oral contraceptives. Use of Lunelle™ was associated with menstrual bleeding lasting more than seven days in 42% of first cycles and 29% of cycles after one year. In addition, 15% of Lunelle™ users had irregular bleed-ing throughout their cycles and 19% developed amenorrhea (1). The average weight gain on Lunelle™ was 4 lbs. after one year. However, a significant number of women gained 10 to 20 lbs. The maximum weight gain was 48 lbs. Also, some women lost weight while using Lunelle™ (25). In a study of women using Lunelle™, cholecystitis and cholelithiasis were the only serious side effects, with a combined incidence of six per 1,000 users (1).

Return to fertility was more rapid after Lunelle™ than following MPA 150. The time to return of ovulation for women using Lunelle™ ranged from 63 to 112 days after the last injection. In women attempting pregnancy after Lunelle™ use, 50% achieved pregnancy within six months and 83% did so within one year (1). Women with lower body weights conceive sooner than women with higher body weights after discontinuing MPA use (1). The effect of Lunelle™ on the fetus and lactation should be assumed to be the same as for MPA 150 users if Lunelle™ is continued during pregnancy. Therefore it is imperative that women who develop amenorrhea should have a urine pregnancy test before their monthly injection.

Breast cancer risk information for Lunelle™ users was not supplied in the physician package information. In the absence of other information the risk of breast cancer in women who used Lunelle™ must be assumed to be increased and the same as for MPA150 (see above).

References for Section 13: Injected Contraceptives

1. Depo-Provera®, Lunelle™, Mirena®, NuvaRing®, Ortho-Evra® package inserts.
2. Smit J, Botha J, McFadyen L, Beksinska M. Serum medroxy-progesterone acetate levels in new and repeated users of depot medroxyprogesterone acetate at the end of the dosing interval. Contraception 2004;69:3–7.
3. Petta Carlos A et al.: Timing of onset of contraceptive effectiveness in Depo-Provera users: Part II. Effects on ovarian function. Fertil Steril 1998;70(5):817–820.
4. Villanueva Gasca A, Bravo Sandoval J: Mechanism of action of a new injectable hormonal contraceptive [translation]. Medicina Rev Mex 1975;55(1194):65–70.
5. Petta Carlos A et al.: Timing of onset of contraceptive effectiveness in Depo-Provera users: Part I. Changes in cervical mucus. Fertil Steril 1998;69(2):252–257.

6. Zeron Medina F: Fertility regulation and some side effects of the use of combined medroxyprogesterone acetate and estradiol cypionate [translation]. Medicina Rev Mex 1974;54(1184):339–345.

7. Schwallie PC, Assenzo JH: Contraceptive use-efficacy study utilizing medroxyprogesterone acetate administered as an intramuscular injection once every 90 days. Fertil Steril 1973;24:331–339.

8. Gongsakdi D, Rojanasakul A: Galactorrhea in DMPA users: Incidence and clinical significance. J Med Assoc Thai 1986;69(1): 28–32.

9. Cundy T, Cornish J, Roberts , Reid IR. Menopausal bone loss in long-term users of medroxyprogesterone acetate contraception. Am J Obstet Gynecol 2002;186:978–83.

10. Deslypere JP, Thiery M, Vermeulen A: Effect of long-term hormonal contraception on plasma lipids. Contraception 1985;31(6): 633–642.

11. Van Deijk WA, Biljham GH, Mellink WAM, Meulenberg PMM: Influence of aminoglutethimide on plasma levels of medroxyprogesterone acetate: Its correlation with serum cortisol. Cancer Treatment Rep. 1985;69:85–90.

12. Westhoff Carolyn et al.: Depressive symptoms and Norplant® contraceptive implants. Contraception 1998;57:241–245.

13. World Health Organization Collaborative Study of Cardiovascular Disease and Steroid Hormone Contraception. Cardiovascular disease and use of oral and injectable progestogen-only contraceptives and combined injectable contraceptives. Contraception 1998;57:315–324.

14. Skegg, DCG, Noonan EA, Paul C, Spears GFS, Meirik O, Thomas DB: Depot medroxyprogesterone acetate and breast cancer: A pooled analysis from the World Health Organization and New Zealand studies. JAMA 1995;273:799–804.

15. World Health Organization (WHO) Collaborative Study of Neoplasia and Steroid Contraceptives. Breast cancer and depomedroxyprogesterone acetate: A multinational study. Lancet 1991; 338:833–838.

16. World Health Organization (WHO) Collaborative Study of Neoplasia and Steroid Contraceptives. Depomedroxyprogesterone acetate (DMPA) and risk of invasive squamous cell cervical cancer. Contraception 1992;45:299–312.

17. World Health Organization (WHO) Collaborative Study of Neoplasia and Steroid Contraceptives. Depomedroxyprogesterone acetate (DMPA) and risk of endometrial cancer. Int J Cancer 1991;49:186–190.

18. World Health Organization (WHO) Collaborative Study of Neoplasia and Steroid Contraceptives. Depomedroxyprogesterone acetate (DMPA) and risk of epithelial ovarian cancer. Int J Cancer 1991;49:191–95.

19. World Health Organization (WHO) Collaborative Study of Neoplasia and Steroid Contraceptives. Depomedroxyprogesterone acetate (DMPA) and risk of liver cancer. Int J Cancer 1991;49: 182–85.

20. Gray RH, Pardthaisong T: Utero exposure to steroid contraceptives and survival during infancy. Am J Epidermiol. 1991;134: 795–803.

21. Pardthaisong T, Gray RH: In utero exposure to steroid contraceptives and outcome of pregnancy. Am J Epidermiol 1991;134: 795–803.

22. Pardthaisong T, Gray RH, McDaniel EB, Chandacham A: Steroid contraceptive use and pregnancy outcome. Teratology 1988;38:51–58.

23. Jimenez J et al.: Long-term follow-up of children breastfed by mothers receiving depomedroxyprogesterone acetate. Contraception 1984;30(6):523–533.

24. Garza-Flores J et al.: Introduction of Cyclofemä once-a-month injectable contraceptive in Mexico. Contraception 1998;58:7–12.

25. Del Junco DJ et al.: Do oral contraceptives prevent rheumatoid arthritis? JAMA 1985;254(14): 1938–1941.

SECTION 14: VAGINAL CONTRACEPTIVE RING

NuvaRing®
etonogestrel / ethinyl estradiol vaginal ring
(Manufacturer: Organon, Inc.)

Description

The etonogestrel-releasing vaginal ring NuvaRing® is a non-biodegradable, flexible, transparent, colorless, combination contraceptive vaginal ring containing 11.7 mg. Etonogestrel, the active metabolite of desogestrel, and 2.7 mg of ethinyl estradiol. When placed in the vagina, each ring releases on average 0.120 mg (120 µg) per day of etonogestrel and 0.015 mg (15 µg) per day of ethinyl estradiol, for three weeks. Bioavailability of etonogestrel after vaginal administration is approximately 100%. Bioavailability of ethinyl estradiol after vaginal administration is approximately 55%. The ovulation inhibiting dosage of etonogestrel is 60 µg/day (1). NuvaRing® is made of ethylene vinylacetate copolymers and magnesium stearate. It has an outer diameter of 54 mm and a cross-sectional diameter of 4mm.

Clinical Information

The NuvaRing® is designed to provide contraception for three weeks when placed in the vagina after which it should be removed for seven days, during which a withdrawal bleed should occur. However, it may remain an effective contraceptive for at least one additional week, allowing a grace period for replacement. A new ring is inserted seven days after the last ring was removed (1). The pregnancy rate for the Nuva-Ring® is <1 per 100 women years in clinical use (2).

NuvaRing® is a combination hormonal contraceptive. As such, it may cause any or all of the minor and serious side effects, and it has the same contraindications to use as contraceptive pills. There is no epidemiological data available to determine whether safety and efficacy with the vaginal route of administration of combination hormonal contraceptives would be different from the oral route. Although no cases of venous thrombosis are listed in the physician package of information, some cases have been reported to the manufacturer.

Practitioners prescribing NuvaRing® should be familiar with the side effects and contraindications of oral contraceptive use. NuvaRing® may not be suitable for women with conditions that make the vagina more susceptible to vaginal irritation or ulceration. Concurrent use of vaginal miconazole increases serum levels of etonogestrel and ethinyl estradiol by 15 to 16%.

Side effects reported by 5 to 14% of women using NuvaRing® include vaginitis, leucorrhoea, weight gain, nausea, headache, sinusitis and upper respiratory infection. Between 1 and 2.5% of women in clinical trials discontinue NuvaRing® due to these symptoms or to other symptoms including: foreign body sensation, coital problems, or device expulsion (1). In US and Canadian studies breakthrough bleeding and spotting occurred in 7.2 to 11.7% of cycles and absence of withdrawal bleeding occurred in 2.3 to 3.8% of cycles. These rates were approximately half as high in European studies (2). Some women experienced amenorrhea or oligomenorrhea after discontinuing NuvaRing®, especially when such conditions were pre-existent.

Management

In patients who did not use hormonal contraception during the previous month, NuvaRing® should be inserted on or prior to day five of the cycle, even if the patient has not finished bleeding. Additional methods of contraception such as condoms or spermicide should be used for the first seven days after insertion. If a combination OC, or the NuvaRing®, has been used in the previous month, NuvaRing® should be inserted no later than day seven of the cycle, even if bleeding has not finished. In patients switching from progestin only OCs, contraceptive implants, or progestin containing UDS, NuvaRing® should be inserted the day the previous method is discontinued, and additional methods of contraception such as condoms or spermicide should be used for the first seven days after insertion. NuvaRing® may be inserted five days following a first trimester abortion or ectopic pregnancy. NuvaRing® may be inserted four weeks following a term pregnancy in women who do not breast feed. Women who are breast feeding should be advised not to use NuvaRing® until the child is weaned.

If NuvaRing® has been removed or expelled during the three week use period it should be rinsed in warm (not hot) water and reinserted within 3 hours. If the ring has been out of the vagina for more than 3 hours, additional methods of contraception must be used for seven days. If menstruation does not occur during the seven days after the ring is removed a pregnancy test must be performed.

Breakthrough bleeding (BTB) and spotting may occur during the three weeks of NuvaRing® use. If abnormal bleeding persists, is severe, or accompanied by pain, appropriate investigation should be instituted to rule out the possibility of organic pathology, pregnancy, or pelvic infection.

The NuvaRing® should not be reused. A new ring must be inserted each month. NuvaRing® may be stored for up to 4 months at 77 °F (25 °C) permissible range 56–86 °F (15–30 °C). It should not be stored in direct sunlight or at temperatures above 86 °F (30 °C).

References For Section 14: Vaginal Ring Contraceptive

1. NuvaRing® package insert.
2. Roumen FJME, Apter D, Mulders TMT, Dieben TOM. Efficacy, tolerability and acceptability of a novel contraceptive vaginal ring releasing etonogestrel and ethinyl estradiol. Hum Reprod 2001;16:469–75.

NOTES

SECTION 15:
CONTRACEPTIVE PATCH

Ortho-Evra®
norelgestromin / ethinyl estradiol
(Ortho-McNeil Pharmaceutical)

The Ortho-Evra® contraceptive patch contains 6 mg of norelgestromin and 0.75 mg ethinyl estradiol (EE). It has a contact surface area of 20 cm². Norelgestromin is the primary active metabolite produced following oral administration, serum levels of norelgestromin are 40 times those of norgestimate (1). Human endometrial receptor binding affinities of norelgestromin are 10 times higher than for norgestimate (2). Each patch releases on average 0.150 mg (150 µg) of norelgestromin and 0.020 mg (20µg) of EE per day for three weeks. Following application of Ortho-Evra®, serum levels reach a constant state in approximately 48 hours of 0.6 to 0.8 µg/ml for norelgestromin and 40 to 50 µg/ml for EE (3). These levels are within the reference ranges for norelgestromin (0.6 to 1.2 µg/ml) and EE (25 to 75 µg/ml) observed in subjects taking a combination OC containing 0.25 mg (250 µg) norgestimate and 0.035 mg (35 µg) EE. Following removal, serum levels of norelgestromin remain elevated for 36 hours (1). During patch replacement, serum levels of norelgestromin and EE drop slightly during the first six hours but remain within the reference range and recover within 12 hours.

Ortho-Evra® consists of three layers. The backing layer is composed of a beige-colored flexible low-density polyethylene. The middle layer contains norelgestromin/polybutene adhesive, crospovidone, non-woven polyester fabric and lauryl lactate. The third layer is a transparent polyethylene terphthalate film that protects the adhesive layer during storage and is removed immediately prior to application. The outside of the backing layer is heat-stamped "ORTHO EVERA® 150/20".

As Ortho-Evra® is applied transdermally, first-pass metabolism (via the gastrointestinal tract and liver) is avoided. Norelgestromin is primarily bound to albumin and

15.

80

not to SHBG, in comparison to norgestrel, which is primarily bound to SHBG.

Clinical Information

Each Ortho-Evra® patch is designed to provide contraception for seven days, after which it is replaced for a second and third week, followed by a rest period of seven days, during which a withdrawal bleed should occur. Only one patch should be worn at a time. If more than seven days pass without the patch being replaced, additional contraceptive measures must be used. Under conditions encountered in a heath club (sauna, whirlpool and treadmill), the serum level of norelgestromin was unaffected while absorption of EE was slightly increased.

The pregnancy rate for the Ortho-Evra® is one per 100 women years of use. However, in clinical studies, pregnancy rates were significantly higher (nine per 100 women years of use) in women who weighed 198 lbs. (90 kg) or more.

The Ortho-Evra® patch is a combination hormonal contraceptive. As such, it may cause any or all of the minor or serious side effects, and it has the same contraindications to use as oral contraceptive pills. There is no epidemiological data available to determine whether safety and efficacy with the transdermal route of administration of combination hormonal contraceptives would be different from the oral route. In clinical trials one case of non-fatal pulmonary embolism occurred during and one case following 1,704 women years of use.

Side effects reported by 9 to 22% of 3,330 women during clinical trials of Ortho-Evra® include in decreasing order of incidence: breast symptoms, headache, application site reaction, nausea, upper respiratory infection, menstrual cramps and abdominal pain. Between 1 and 2.4% of women in clinical trials discontinued Ortho-Evra®. The most frequent causes of discontinuation were nausea, application site reaction, breast symptoms, headache and emotional labiality.

In clinical trials, most women started withdrawal bleeding on the fourth drug-free day, whereas following OC pills most women experience bleeding on the second post pill day.

The median duration of bleeding was five to six days. In 26% of cycles, breakthrough bleeding or spotting lasted several days (this included withdrawal bleeding).

Following discontinuation, FSH, LHL, and estradiol may not return to baseline values until six weeks or later. Fertility may be decreased during this period. Ortho-Evra® is rated pregnancy Category X. In rabbits, at doses 25 to 125 times human doses, paw hyperflexion and cleft palate were noted. Ortho-Evra® should be removed immediately if pregnancy occurs.

Management

Patients using Ortho-Evra® for the first time should apply the patch on the first day of their menstrual period. Patients who choose to start after the first day (e.g., Sunday start) should use additional contraception, such as condoms or spermicide, for the first seven days.

The Ortho-Evra® patch should be started no earlier than four weeks following a term pregnancy. The patch should not be used by women who are breastfeeding. The patch may be started immediately following a first trimester abortion or ectopic pregnancy. If the patch is started more than four days following a first trimester abortion, additional contraceptive methods should be used.

The patch should be applied to clean, dry skin on the buttock, abdomen, upper arm or upper torso in a place where it will not be rubbed by clothing. The patch should not be applied to red or irritated skin, nor should it be placed on the breasts. If patch use results in irritation, the patch should be removed and a new patch applied to a different location.

Target levels of norelgestromin and EE are maintained during an eighth or ninth day of extended use. If a patient forgets to change her patch for more than two days (wears her patch longer than nine days), a new four-week cycle should be started and additional contraception should be used the first seven days.

During clinical trials 4.7% of patches either fell off (1.8%) or were partly detached (2.9%). If a patch is partially or completely detached for less than 24 hours, it should be reapplied or replaced immediately. No additional contraception method is needed. If a patch is partially or completely detached for more than 24 hours, a new four-week cycle should be started and additional contraceptive methods should be used for the first seven days.

Breakthrough bleeding (BTB) or spotting may occur during early cycles of Ortho-Evra® use. If abnormal bleeding persists, is severe, or is accompanied by pain, appropriate investigation should be instituted to rule out the possibility of organic pathology, pregnancy or pelvic infection. If withdrawal bleeding does not occur during the seven patch-free days a pregnancy test should be performed before starting the next patch cycle. An ultrasound test will help to determine whether abnormal bleeding is due to an endometrium that is too thin, indicating insufficient estrogen, or too thick, indicating excessive estrogen effect. In the latter case, an endometrial biopsy is indicated if the endometrial thickness if greater than 10 mm or is uneven. Oral contraceptive pills and progestins should not be used to treat irregular bleeding or amenorrhea that may occur while using the Ortho-Evra® patch.

References for Section 15: Contraceptive Patch

1. McGuire JL, Phillips A, Hahn DW, Tolman EL, Flor S, Kafrissen ME: Pharmacologic and pharmacokinetic characteristics of norgestimate. Amer J Obstet Gynecol 1990;47:2127–2131.
2. Juchem M, Pollow E, Elger W, Hoffman G, Mobus V: Receptor binding of norgestimate: A new orally active synthetic progestational compound. Contraception 1993;47:283–294.
3. Depo-Provera®, Lunelle™, Mirena®, NuvaRing®, Ortho-Evra® package inserts.

SECTION 16: PROGESTIN-FILLED INTRAUTERINE DELIVERY SYSTEM

Mirena®
levonorgestrel-releasing intrauterine system
(Berlex Lab INC)

Description

The levonorgestrel-releasing (LNG 20) intrauterine device, manufactured in Finland, has been used extensively in Europe since 1990. The LNG 20 has the same polyethylene skeleton as the Paragard® copper-wrapped IUD. The progestin is homogeneously dispersed in a polydimethylsiloxane reservoir covered by a rate-limiting membrane on the vertical arm of the device. The initial *in vitro* release rate of LNG is 20 micrograms/24 hours and about 15 micrograms/24 hours after five years. The insertion tube of the LNG 20 IUD is 4.8 mm compared to about 3.8 mm for the copper-wrapped IUD.

Clinical Information

The LNG 20 IUD is designed for five years use, after which it should be replaced. However, it may remain an effective contraceptive for at least 18 additional months, allowing a grace period for replacement. The annual and five year cumulative pregnancy rates for LNG 20 IUD are 0.1 and 0.5%; respectively, approximately 10 times lower than for copper-wrapped IUDs. If pregrancy does occur, as many as 50% of pregnancies will be ectopic (1, 2, 3). If uterine perforation occurs, the LNG IUD should be retrieved from the peritoneal cavity as soon as possible. Serum levels of LNG are increased 10-fold when an LNG IUD is located intra-peritoneal (4).

The local effect of LNG in the uterine cavity causes reduction of menstrual blood loss and development of oligoamenorrhea. As a result, termination rates because of heavy and/or prolonged menstrual flow are significantly reduced compared to copper-wrapped IUDS; hemoglobin rates rise slightly during prolonged use. Changes in the men-

16.

84

strual bleeding pattern are common but are well accepted by most women (5, 6, 7, 8). Amenorrhea develops in 20% of LNG users by one year (9). The proportion of women reporting menstrual pain was reduced from 60% before using Mirena® to 29% after 36 months of use in one study (5).

The cumulative five-year incidence of pelvic inflammatory disease (PID) requiring removal of the LNG 20 IUD was 0.8% compared to 2.2% for copper-wrapped IUDs. The difference was most marked in women ages 25 years and younger for whom the termination rate for PID was 0.3% for LNG 20 compared to 5.6% for copper-wrapped IUDs (7).

Hormonal effects and other effects at three months of use included:

- Low abdominal pain—10.5%
- Acne—3.5%
- Mastalgia—3.1%
- Headache—2.8%
- Depression—2.5%
- Nausea—2.4%.

All were higher for the LNG 20 IUD than for a copper-wrapped IUD at three months, but there was no difference after 60 months. Ovarian cysts occurred in 12% of LNG 20 IUD users (9).

After removal of the LNG 20, women who wanted to become pregnant did so within 12 months.

Management

The LNG 20 may be somewhat more difficult to insert than copper-wrapped IUDs due to their larger diameter. This was particularly noted at the time of second and third insertions. IUDs should not be inserted post partum until uterine involution has occurred. Serum LNG levels in nursing infants were 7% of mothers' levels in women who had LNG 20 IUDs inserted while nursing. The LNG 20 IUD should be removed immediately if pregnancy occurs, due to the androgen and progestational activities of LNG. In 32 live births following LNLG 20 IUD exposure, there were two birth defects, one pulmonary artery hypoplasia, possibly related to progestin use.

Infection

IUDs shold be removed immediately and antibiotic treatment initiated if endometriosis or PID are diagnosed. Actinomycosis is associated with IUD use. The symptoms of PID include prolonged heavy bleeding, unusual discharge, dyspareunia, pelvic pain, chills and fever. Endometriosis severe enough to cause tubal damage may also be asymptomatic.

Contraindications

IUD use is contraindicated in women with congenital or acquired uterine anomaly, including fibroids if they distort the uterine cavity, acute PID or a history of PID unless there has been a subsequent intrauterine pregnancy, postpartum endometriosis or insertion is within three months following an infected abortion, multiple sexual partners, untreated cervicitis or vaginal infection, vaginal bleeding of unknown cause, uterine or cervical cancer and conditions associated with increased susceptibility to infection with microorganisms, including leukemia and acquired immunodeficiency syndrome (AIDS).

References for Section 16: Progestin-filled Intrauterine Device

1. Kubba AAC, Guillebud J: Case of ectopicpregnancy after post-coital contraception with ethinyl oestradiol-LNG. Br Med J 1983;287:1343. 230 231
2. Ory HW and the Women's Health Study: Ectopic pregnancy and intrauterine contraceptive devices. Am J Obstet Gynecol 1981; 57:137.
3. Backman T, Rauramo I, Huhtala S, Koskenvuo M. Pregnancy during use of levonorgestrel intrauterine system. Am J Obstet Gynecol 2004;190:50–4.
4. Haimov-Kochman R, Amsalem H, Adoni A, Lavy Y, M.Spitz I. Management of a perforated levonorgestrel-medicated intrauterine

device-a pharmacokinetic study: Case report. Hum Reprod 2003;18:1232–3.

5. Baldaszti E, Wimmer-Puchinger B, Löschke K. Acceptability of the long-term contraceptive levonorgestrel-releasing intrauterine system (Mirena®): a 3-year follow-up study. Contreception 2003; 7:87–91.

6. French RS, Cowan FM, Maansour D, et al. Levonorgestrel-releasing (20ug/day) intrauterine systems (Mirena) compared with other methods of reversible contraceptives. Br J Obstet Gynaecol 2000;107:1218–25.

7. Anderson K, Odlind V, Rybo G. Levonorgestrel-releasing and copper releasing (Nova-T) intrauterine devices during five years of use: a randomized comparative trial. Contreception 1994;49:56–72.

8. Suvisaari J, Lahteenmaki P. Detailed analysis of menstrual bleeding patterns after postmenstrual and postabortal insertion of a copper IUI or a levonorgestrel-releasing intrauterine system. Contreception 1996;54:201–8.

9. Depo-Provera®, Lunelle™, Mirena®, NuvaRing®, Ortho-Evra® package inserts.

SECTION 17: IMPLANTS AND DEVELOPMENTAL CONTRACEPTIVES

Norplant®—Norplant I

Status

Norplant I was released for general use in the United States after study since 1980. Use was low and was accompanied by lawsuits due to side effects primarily related to irregular bleeding and difficulty of removal. A survey in 1995 found that 0.9% of American women age 15 to 44 had an implant (Norplant I) compared to 17.3% who were using OCs. In late August 2000 sale was suspended in the United States because of manufacturing problems resulting in low levels of drug release. The manufacturer, Wyeth, has stated that it will not reintroduce Norplant in the United States but it may continue to be available in other countries (Ob. Gyn News September 1, 2002).

Management and Dose

Norplant I implants contained 36 mg Levonorgestrel (LNG) per Silastic® capsule. Six LNG capsules, each measuring 2.4 by 34 mm, were implanted, with a 10-gauge trocar, subdermally in a fan-like pattern through a 3 to 5 mm incision in the medial aspect of the upper, volar side of the forearm.

Insertions were made during the first seven days after onset of menstruation. Insertions can also be made immediately postpartum in nonnursing women and postabortion.

Onset of Contraception

The primary contraceptive action may be impairment of embryo of implantation. Changes in cervical mucus and sperm penetration are evident 24 hours after insertion of implants. However, additional contraception (e.g., condoms or contraceptive foam) should be used until 72 hours after insertion (1). LNG was identified in the breast milk of Norplant I users (2), therefore LNG implants are not recommended for breastfeeding women.

17.

Removal

Removal, performed under local anesthesia, was through a small incision. Removal may be difficult if capsules are inserted too deeply. Nonpalpable capsules could be located by ultrasound.

Complications were reported in 4.5% of implant removals in a multinational study (3). Most complications during removal were related to broken or deeply imbedded implants (3).

Capsules were intended to be removed or replaced after five years (after two years in women who weigh more than 70 kg [154 lbs.]) since effectiveness decreases after that time. However, no harmful effects occured if capsules were not removed unless a patient became pregnant. Spontaneous expulsion occurred in the presence of infection and when insertions were too close to the incision.

Capsules must be removed immediately if pregnancy occurs due to the potential masculinizing effect of NG.

Contraindications

Contraindications were the same as for OCs.

Clinical Information

Norplant I had a cumulative pregnancy rate of 3.9 per 100 women after five years, an average of 0.8% failures per year (4). The rate of release of LNG depends in part on body fat and blood supply in the area of implantation. Plasma levels of LNG are inversely related to body weight. In women who weighed 145 lbs. (70 kg) or more, pregnancy rates were 5.1 per 100 women in the third year of use and 8.5 after five years. A study of Chinese women found a similar relationship to weight, but cumulative five-year pregnancy rates were only half as high (5).

Ectopic Pregnancy

The incidence of ectopic pregnancy in Norplant I users was 1.3 per 1,000 women years (4). This is less than the 2.3 to 3.0 per 1,000 women years reported to occur in the general population.

Any Norplant I patient who presents with lower abdominal pain must be evaluated to rule out ectopic pregnancy.

Bleeding Irregularities

Implants, like other progestin-only contraceptives, disrupt the menstrual cycle.

One study reported disruption of the menstrual cycle in 60 to 80% of users in the first year (6). The FDA-approved package insert reported irregular or prolonged bleeding and/or spotting in 58% of Norplant I users during the first year of use (4). In other studies, 36% of patients experienced irregular bleeding during the first three months; during the ninth to twelfth months, only 12% experienced irregular bleeding. Despite the bleeding, total average menstrual blood loss was less than before treatment, and Hg/HCT levels rose during use (7, 8, 9). An analysis of patients with irregular bleeding found that they had low estradiol levels, absence of luteal activity, and a thin hyperecogenic pattern in the endometrium (10).

Amenorrhea

The FDA-approved package insert reported amenorrhea in 9.4% and scant menses in 5.2% of users (2).

In other studies, amenorrhea lasting more than 60 days occurred in 32% of patients during the first three months and in 24% during the ninth to 12th months (9, 11). Therefore, missed menstrual periods cannot serve as the only means of identifying early pregnancy. Pregnancy tests should be performed whenever a pregnancy is suspected. If pregnancy occurs, the capsules must be removed.

Ovarian Cysts

In seven new drug application clinical trials, temporary enlargement of the fallopian tubes and ovarian (follicular) cysts occurred in 0.8 to 4.6% and abdominal pain occurred in 1.7 to 8.7% of Norplant I users during the first year of use (2). In the majority of women, enlarged follicular cysts disappeared spontaneously and did not require surgery.

Idiopathic Intracranial Hypertension

Thirty-nine cases of idiopathic intracranial hypertension (pseudotumor cerebri) had been reported in Norplant I users as of 1993 (5.5 cases per 100,00 vs the expected incidence of 3.5 cases per 100,000) (12). Pseudotumor is characterized by papilledema and unremitting headache. If pseudotumor is confirmed, Norplant® implants should be removed.

Cardiovascular Effects

Superficial thrombophlebitis in the arm of insertion has been reported. There were 14 hospitalizations for stroke in a 1995 review of serious events in Norplant I users (13). A subsequent case-control analysis found that the relative risk of stroke and acute myocardial infarction were not increased compared with the general population of women (14).

Other Serious Side Effects

Between the time of the introduction of implants in the U.S. in February 1991 and December 1993, the FDA received 5,800 reports of adverse events in implant users, of which 100 were serious (13). The serious events included: 24 hospitalizations for infection at the insertion site, 14 reports of patients disabled because of difficult implant removal, 14 cases of stroke, 6 cases of thrombotic thrombocytopenia or thrombocytopenia purpura, 39 cases of pseudotumor cerebri, of which 11 required hospitalization.

Laboratory Changes

Both increases and decreases in high-density lipoprotein- (HDL) cholesterol levels were reported in clinical trials (see manufacturer package insert or physician information). No statically significant increases were reported in the ratio of total cholesterol-to-HDL-cholesterol. Low-density lipoprotein (LDL)-cholesterol and triglyceride levels were decreased during Norplant I use (2). Blood glucose levels were shown to be elevated but within normal range. Coagulation studies showed a small increase in factor VII and a decrease in antithrombin III (2).

Drug Interactions

Reduced efficacy was reported in Norplant® users taking phenytoin and carbamazine (2).

Other Clinical Information

The contraceptive effect of Norplant I is reversed by removal of the implants; 77% of users became pregnant within the first year after removal (4). The time to conception was not affected by duration of use (2).

DEVELOPMENTAL CONTRACEPTIVES

Norplant II (Jadell)

Contraceptive implants, made of flexible nonbiodegradable tubes filled with hormones and placed under the skin, were first developed in the 1960s. At least 10 compounds have been tested in implants. Currently, other Silastic® and biodegradeable implants are under investigation.

Norplant II or Jadelle is the only other implant approved by the FDA. Norplant II consists of two rods, compared to six for Norplant I, each measuring 0.25 cm diameter and 4.3 cm in length, about 1 cm longer than Norpland I rods. Jadell contains 75 mg of levonorgestrel in each rod for a total of 150 mg. Jadell releases levonorgestrel at a rate of 80 µg per day in the first month, with a gradual decrease to 25–30 µg per day after the 9th month. In clinical trials in the US it was as effective as Norplant I and required an average of two minutes to insert and 4.5 minutes to remove (15). Jadell was approved by the FDA for 3-year use in 1999, and approval was extended to allow use for 5 years in 2001. Despite approval, the manufacturer, Wyeth, has not released Jadell for sale in the United States. If Jadell is released, use and management of side effects are expected to be the same as for Norplant I.

Injections

Norethindrone enanthate (Schering), the heptanoic acid ester of norethindrone, has been tested extensively in World

Health Organization (WHO) studies for use in injections since the early 1970s. There are no current plans for its release in the U.S.

Gonadotrophin-releasing Hormone Injections

Gonadotrophin-releasing hormone (GnRH) injections have been under investigation for many years (16). GnRH agonists, given monthly, are effective in suppressing ovulation (17). Long-term use for contraception is not recommended due to a propensity of GnRH to cause bone loss.

Male Contraception

Although trials of hormonal and nonhormonal male contraceptive pills and injections have been conducted for many years, none are near release for clinical use (18, 19, 20). A 2003 review summarizes the reasons (21).

Spermatogenesis, male body characteristics, and the male sex act depend on the presence of male hormones, principally testosterone. Attempts to suppress active testosterone or the pituitary gonadotropins in order to prevent spermatogenesis inevitably alter the male sexual response and male body characteristics. Sperm concentration must be suppressed to < 3 million per ml for effectiveness in 99% of men. Past and recent studies performed on Asian men in Asia and the United States revealed that hormonal regimens found effective in Asia were less effective in Western men (21).

Significant side effects of androgens include liver and prostate cancers and cardiovascular disease. Other side effects are acne, weight gain, and effect on hemoglobin and lipid levels.

One proven method of male hormone contraception, at least in Asian men, is monthly injection of testosterone undecanoate (22). Recent studies have involved combining long-acting delivery systems effective in women with traditional methods of effective testosterone administration. These include testosterone implants every 4 to 6 months combined with medroxyprogesterone acetate (MPA) every 3 months (23), and LGN combined with transdermal and injectable testosterone (24). MPA injection has been used for male sex offenders to inhibit libido (25). GnRH analogs with testosterone to counteract impotence have also been investigated but there was concern about osteoporosis.

An important deterent to male hormonal contraception remains the need for monthly injections.

GOSSYPOL

Gossypol, a polyphenol derivative of cottonseed similar to flavonoids taken orally daily, is 99% effective for male contraception after two to three months of use. Fertility returns after six months to three years. Gossypol is well tolerated causing no side effects that lead to discontinuation. Reported hypokalemia of early studies has not been confirmed in later trials, Permanent sterility occurs in 10 to 20% of patients (11, 26). Therefore Gossypol use should be limited to men who have completed their families.

References for Section 17: Implants and Developmental Contraceptives

1. Dunn NR, Thorogood M, de Caestecker L, Mann RD: Myocardial infarction and oral contraceptives: A retrospective case-control study in England and Scotland (MICA study). Pharmacoepidemiol Drug Safety 1997;6:283–289.
2. Norplant® package insert. Wyeth Laboratories, Inc., December 11, 1998.
3. Dunson Thomas R et al.: Timing of onset of contraceptive effectiveness in Norplant® implant users: Part I. Changes in cervical mucus. Fertil Steril 1998;69(2):258–266.
4. Nattero G: Menstrual headache. Adv Neurol 1982;33:215–226.
5. Spitzer WO, Lewis MA, Heinemann LAJ, Thorogood M, MacRae KD: Third-generation oral contraceptives and risk of venous thromboembolic disorders: An international case control study. BMJ 1996;312:83–87.
6. Shikary ZK, Betrabet SS, Patel ZM, et al.: Transfer of LNG administered through different drug delivery systems from the maternal circulation into newborn infant's circulation. Contraception 1987; 35:477–486.
7. Phillips et al.: Comprehensive comparison of the potencies and activities of progestogens used in contraceptives. Contraception 1987;36:181.

8. Thomsen RJ: Utilization of Norplant® subdermal contraceptive devices. Clin Obstet 1985; 23(3):223–227.

9. World Health Organization (WHO): Facts about an implantable contraceptive. Memorandum. Bull WHO 1985;63(3):485–494.

10. Kaewrudee S, Taneepanichskul S. Norplant® users with irregular bleeding. J Reprod Med 2000;45:983–6.

11. Population Information Program. Population Reports. Series A, No. 2, 1975; Series H, No. 2, May 1974; Series I, No. 1, June 1974; Series B, No. 2, January 1976. Washington, DC: George Washington University Medical Center.

12. Wynn V: Effect of duration of low-dose oral contraceptive administration on carbohydrate metabolism. Am J Obstet Gynecol 1982;142:739.

13. Wysowski DK, Green L: Serious adverse events in Norplant® users reported to the Food and Drug Administration's MedWatch Spontaneous Reporting System. Obstet Gynecol 1995;85:538–542.

14. Petitti Diana B et al.: Norplant® implants and cardiovascular disease. Contraception 1998;57:361–362.

15. Wan LS, Stiber A, Lam L. The levonorgestrel two-rod implant for long-acting contraception: 10 years of clinical experience. Obstet Gynecol 2003;102:24–6.

16. Swyer GIM, Little V: Clinical assessment of relative potency of progestogens. J Repro Fertil 1968;5(suppl):63–68.

17. Brinton LA et al.: Long-term use of oral contraceptives and risk of invasive cervical cancer. Int J Cancer 1986;38(3):339–344.

18. Dickey RP, Stone SC: Progestational potency of oral contraceptives. Am J Obstet Gynecol 1976;47:106–111.

19. Diczfalusy E: New developments in oral, injectable, and implantable contraceptives, vaginal rings, and intrauterine devices: A review. Contraception 1986;33(1):7–22.

20. Nissen ED, Kent DR, Nissen SE: Etiologic factors in the pathogenesis of liver tumors associated with oral contraceptives. Am J Obstet Gynecol 1977;127:61.

21. Handelsman DJ. Editorial: Hormonal male contraception-Lessons from the East when the Western market fails. J Clin Endocrinol Metab 2003;88:599–61.

22. Gu Y-Q, Wang X-H, Xu D, Peng L, Cheng L-F, Huang M-K, Hung Z-J, Zhang G-Y. A multicenter contraceptive Efficacy study of injectable testosterone undecanoate in healthy Chinese men. J Clin Endocrinol Metab 2003;88:562–8.

23. Turner l, Conway AJ, Jimenez M, Liu P, Forbes E, McLachlan RI, Handelsman DJ. Contraceptive efficacy of a depot progestin and androgen combination in men. J Clin Endocrinol Metab 2003; 88:5659–67.

24. Gonzalo ITG, Swerdloff RS, Nelson AL, Clevenger B, Garcia R, Berman N, Wang C. Levonorgestrel implants (Norplant II) for male contraception clinical trialsL Combination with transdermal and injectable testosterone. J Clin Endocrinol Metab 2003;88:3562–72.

25. Fregly MJ, Thrasher TN: Response of heart rate to acute administration of isoproterenol in rats treated chronically with norethynodrel, EE, and both combined. Endocrinology 1977;100(1):148–154.

26. Coutinho EM. Gossypol: a contraceptive for men. Contraception 2002;65:259–63.

NOTES

SECTION 18: TABLES

TABLE 1: BENEFICIAL EFFECTS OF ORAL CONTRACEPTIVES

Condition or Disease	Percent Reduction Compared to Nonusers	References
Pregnancy		
Term vaginal delivery	99	1
Term cesarean section	99	1
Spontaneous abortion, D & C	99	1
Ectopic pregnancy	99	1
Menstrual Disorders		
Dysmenorrhea	63	2
Menopausal symptoms	72	2
Menorrhagia	48	2
Irregular menstruation	35	2
Intermenstrual bleeding	28	2
Premenstrual tension	29	2
Reproductive Organ Neoplasm		
Fibrocystic and fibroadenoma breast disease	50 to 75	3, 4, 5, 6, 7
Breast biopsies	50	1
Benign ovarian cysts	65	8, 9, 10

Uterine fibroma*	59	2, 8
Ovarian cancer	40	11, 12
Endometrial cancer	50	13, 14, 15, 16, 17, 18, 19
Other Reproductive Disorders		
Endometriosis*	50	2, 8, 20
Pelvic inflammatory disease– all cases*	10 to 70	21
Pelvic inflammatory disease– hospitalized cases*	10 to 70	21
Toxic shock syndrome	60	22
Uterine retroversion	24	2
Other Conditions		
Colorectal Cancer	19	23
Rheumatoid arthritis	50	2, 24, 25
Iron deficiency anemia	45	2, 9, 26
Duodenal ulcer	40	2
Sebaceous cysts	24	2
Acne	16	2

*These conditions may have a significant adverse effect on future reproductive capabilities.

(continued)

99

References for Table 1: Beneficial Effects of Oral Contraceptives

1. Ory HW: The noncontraceptive health benefits from oral contraceptive use. Fam Plann Perspect 1982;14:182.
2. Royal College of General Practitioners. Oral contraceptives and health: An interim report from the oral contraception study of the Royal College of General Practitioners. New York: Pitman, 1974.
3. Brinton LA et al.: Risk factors for benign breast disease. Am J Epidemiol 1981;113:203–214.
4. Ory HW: Health effects of fertility control. In: Contraception: Science, Technology, and Application: Proceedings of a Symposium. Washington, DC: National Academy of Sciences, 1979;110–121.
5. Ory HW: Oral contraceptive use and breast diseases. In: Pharmacology of Steroid Contraceptive Drugs. Garattini S, Berendes HW (ed.) New York: Raven Press, 1977;179–183.
6. Ory HW et al.: Oral contraceptives and reduced risk of benign breast diseases. N Engl J Med 1976;294:419–422.
7. Royal College of General Practitioners Oral Contraceptive Study. Effect on hypertension and benign breast disease of progestogen component in combined oral contraceptives. Lancet 1977;1:624.
8. Chiaffarino Francesca et al.: Oral contraceptive use and benign gynecologic conditions. Contraception 1998;57:11–18.
9. Vessey MP et al.: A long-term follow-up study of women using different methods of contraception: An interim report. J Biosoc Sci 1976;8:373–427.
10. Ylikorkala O: Ovarian cysts and hormonal contraception. Lancet 1977;1:1101–1102.
11. Centers for Disease Control Cancer and Steroid Hormone Study. Oral contraceptive use and the risk of ovarian cancer. JAMA 1983;249:1596–1599.
12. Weiss NS et al.: Incidence of ovarian cancer in relation to use of oral contraceptives. Int J Cancer 1981;28:669–671.
13. Cohen CJ, Deppe G: Endometrial carcinoma and oral contraceptive pills. Am J Obstet Gynecol 1977;49:390–392.

14. Kaufman DW et al.: Decreased risk of endometrial cancer among oral contraceptive users. N Engl J Med 1980;303:1045.

15. Kay CR: Progestogens before and after menopause. Br Med J 1980;281:811–812.

16. Scotlenfeld D, Engle RL Jr: Decreased risk of endometrial cancer among oral contraceptive users. N Engl J Med 1980; 303:1045.

17. Silverberg SG, Makowski EL: Endometrial carcinoma in young women taking oral contraceptive agents. Am J Obstet Gyencol 1975;46:503–506.

18. Silverberg SG, Makowski EL, Roche WD: Endometrial carcinoma in women under 40 years of age: Comparisons of cases in oral contraceptive users and nonusers. Cancer 1977;39:592–598.

19. Weiss NS, Sayvetz TA et al.: Incidence of endometrial cancer in relation to oral contraceptives. N Engl J Med 1980; 302:551.

20. Vessey MP, Villard-MacKintosh L, Painter R: Epidemiology of endometriosis in women attending family planning clinics. Br Med J 1993;306:182–184.

21. Senanayake P, Kramer DG: Contraception and the etiology of PID: New perspectives. Am J Obstet Gynecol 1980;138:852–860.

22. Gray RH: Toxic shock syndrome and oral contraception. Am J Obst Gynecol 1988;156:1038.

23. Fernandez E, La Vecchia C, Balducci A, Chatenoud L, Franceschi S, Negri E. Oral contraceptives and colorectal cancer risk: a meta analysis. Br J Cancer 2001;84:722–7.

24. Linos A et al.: Rheumatoid arthritis and oral contraceptives. Lancet 1978;2:871.

25. Wingrave SJ, Kay CR: Reduction in incidence of rheumatoid arthritis associated with oral contraceptives. Lancet 1978;1:569.

26. Walnut Creek Contraceptive Drug Study. Results of the Walnut Creek Contraceptive Drug Study. J Repro Med 1980; 25(suppl):346.

TABLE 2: EFFECTIVENESS AND MORTALITY OF CONTRACEPTIVE METHODS

Method	Pregnancies Per 100 Women/Years All Ages[1]		Estimated Annual Deaths Due to Contraceptive Method and/or Pregnancy Per 100,000 Women/Years by Age[2]					
	Lowest Expected	Typical	15–19	20–24	25–29	30–34	35–39	40–44
No Contraception	85	85	6	5	7	14	19	22
Surgical Sterilization[3] (Tubal ligation)	0.2	0.4	4	4	4	4	4	4
Combination Oral Contraceptives Non-smokers	0.1	3	1	1	1	2	4	3
Smokers	0.1	3	2	2	2	11	13	59
Progestin-Only Oral Contraceptives	0.5	3	1	1	1	1	1	1
Progestin Injections Medroxyprogesterone acetate (MPA)	0.3	0.3	1	1	1	1	1	1
Progestin Implants Levonorgestrel (LNG)	0.3	0.3	1	1	1	1	1	1
Intrauterine Devices ParaGard® T 380A	0.8	3	1	1	1	1	1	1

Barrier Methods

Diaphragm Cap	6	18	1–2	1–2	1–2	1–4	1–6	1–7
Condoms	2	12	1–3	1–3	1–4	1–7	1–11	1–12
Aerosol foam, jelly, cream, tablets	3	21	1–3	1–3	1–4	1–7	1–11	1–12
Sponge								
Parous women	9	28	1–2	1–2	1–3	1–6	1–8	1–10
Nulliparous women	6	18	1–2	1–2	1–2	1–4	1–6	1–7
Periodic Abstinence (rhythm)	1–9	20	1–2	1–2	1–2	1–4	1–16	1–16

References for Table 2: Effectiveness and Mortality of Contraceptive Methods

1. Trussell J, Hatcher RA, Cates W Jr., Stewart FH, Kost K: A guide to interpreting contraceptive efficacy studies. Obstet Gynecol 1990;76:558–567.

   Trussell J, Kost K: Contraceptive failure in the United States: A critical review of the literature. Stud Fam Plann.

2. Tietze C, Bongaarts V, Schearer B: Mortality associated with the control of fertility. Fam Plann Perspect 1976;8:6–14.

3. Peterson HB et al.: Mortality risk associated with tubal sterilization in the United States. Am J Obstet Gynecol 1982; 143:125.

In a comparative study of 1,437 women using the sponge vs. diaphragm and a study of 1,394 women using the cervical cap vs. diaphragm the 12 months failure rate was diaphragm 5.2 and 6.9%, cervical cap 11.4%, sponge 11.7%. Failure rates increased to 26.4% for the cap and 20% for the sponge among parous users. The failure rate for condoms was estimated at 2.7%. (see Trussel J, Office of Population Research, Princeton University, 1993).

TABLE 3: PREGNANCY AND CONTINUATION RATES

Method	Pregnancy Typical	Pregnancy Ideal Use	Continuation After 1 year
None	85%	85%	100%
Cervical Cap	40%	26%	42%
Sponge	40%	20%	42%
Spermicides	26%	6%	40%
Physiological	25%	3%	63%
Female Condom	21%	5%	56%
Diaphragm	20%	6%	56%
Male Condom	14%	3%	61%
Pill Combination	2%	<1%	71%
Vaginal Ring	2%	<1%	*
Hormonal Patch	2%	<1%	*
IUD Copper	2%	<1%	78%
Injection	1%	<1%	70%
Implant	1%	<1%	88%

*New

Adapted from Hatcher RA, et al, *Contraceptive Technology, 17th Revised Edition*, NY, NY, Irvington Publishers, 1998

104

TABLE 4: BIOLOGICAL ACTIVITY OF ORAL CONTRACEPTIVE COMPONENTS

Class of Compound	Progestational Activity[1]	Estrogenic Activity[2]	Androgenic Activity[3]	Endometrial Activity[4]	Andro:Prog Activity Ratio[5]
Progestins[6]					
19 Nor-Testosterone Progestins					
Estrane					
Norethindrone	1.0	1.0	1.0	1.0	1.0
Norethindrone acetate	1.2	1.5	1.6	0.4	1.3
Ethynodiol diacetate	1.4	3.4	0.6	0.4	0.4
5(10) Estrane					
Norethynodrel	0.3	8.3	0	0	0
Gonane					
Norgestimate	1.3	0	1.9	1.2	1.5
dl-Norgestrel	2.6	0	4.2	2.6	1.6
Levonorgestrel	5.3	0	8.3	5.1	1.6
Desogestrel	9.0	0	3.4	8.7	0.4
Gestodene	12.6	0	8.6	12.6	0.7
Pregnane Progestins					
Other					
Medroxyprogesterone acetate	0.3	0	0	NA	0
Drospirenone	0.5	0	0	NA	0

(continued)

105

TABLE 4: BIOLOGICAL ACTIVITY OF ORAL CONTRACEPTIVE COMPONENTS (Continued)

Class of Compound	Progestational Activity[1]	Estrogenic Activity[2]	Androgenic Activity[3]	Endometrial Activity[4]	Andro:Prog Activity Ratio[5]
Estrogens[7]					
Ethinyl estradiol	0	100	0	0	0
Mestranol	0	67	0	0	0

1. Based on amount required to induce vacuoles in human endometrium [see Cook CL et al.: Pregnancy prophylaxis: Parenteral postcoital estrogen. Obstet Gynecol 1986;67:331]. Desogestrel, gestodene, levonorgestrel and norgestimate based on oral stimulation of endometrium in immature estrogen-primed rabbits relative to levonorgestrel = 5.3 [see Phillips A et al.: Progestational and androgenic receptor binding affinities and in vitro activities of norgestimate and other progestins. Contraception 1990;41:399–410]

2. Comparative potency based on oral rat vaginal epithelium assay. (Norethindrone = 0.2 when ethinyl estradiol = 100 [see Jones RC, Edgren RA: The effects of various steroids on vaginal histology in the rat. Fertil Steril 1973;24:284–291])

3. Comparative potency (oral) based on rat ventral prostate assay (Norethindrone = 1.0 when methyltestosterone = 50. [see Tausk M, de Visser J: International Encyclopedia of Pharmacology and Therapeutics. Ch. 28, Sect. 48, Vol. II. Elmsford, NY: Pergamon Press, 1972]; Levonorgestrel and desogestrel relative to norethindrone = 1.0. [see Kloosterboer HJ, Deckers GHI: Desogestrel: A selective progestogen. Int Proc J 1989;1:26–30]; Norgestimate, relative to levonorgestrel = 8.3. [see Phillips A et al.: Progestational and androgenic receptor binding affinities and in vitro activities of norgestimate and other progestins. Contraception 1990;41:399–410]; and Gestodene relative to levonorgestrel = 8.3 [see Elger WH et al.: Endocrine pharmacological profile of gestodene. Adv Contracept Delivery Systems 1986;2:182–97])

4. Based on estimation of amount required to suppress bleeding for 20 days in 50% of women [see Swyer GIM, Little V: Potency of progestogens and oral contraceptives: Further delay-of-menses date. Contraception 1982;26:23]

5. Androgenic ÷ progestational activity, based on oral and animal assays. Actual activity in women may be different and will be modified by the dose of estrogen.

6. Calculated on the basis of norethindrone = 1.0 in activity

7. Calculated on the basis of ethinyl estradiol = 100 in activity

TABLE 5: COMPOSITION AND IDENTIFICATION OF ORAL CONTRACEPTIVES

Name	Progestin	mg/tablet	Estrogen	mcg/tablet	Manufacturer	Color A/IA[5,6]	Inactive Ingredient[9]
Monophasic							
Alesse	Levonorgestrel	0.1	E. estradiol[3]	20	Wyeth	P (LG)	d
Apri	Desogestrel	0.15	E. estradiol	30	Barr	Ro(W)	k
Aviane	Levonorgestrel	0.1	E. estradiol[3]	20	Barr	O(LG)	k
Brevicon	Norethindrone	0.5	E. estradiol	35	Watson	Bl (O)	a
Cryselle	Norgestrel	0.3	E. estradiol	30	Barr	W(LG)	i
Demulen 1/35	Ethy. diacetate	1.0	E. estradiol	35	Watson	W (Bl)	b
Demulen 1/50	Ethy. diacetate[1]	1.0	E. estradiol	50	Watson	W (P)	b
Desogen	Desogestrel	0.15	E. estradiol	30	Organon	W (G)	c
Kariva	Desogestrel	0.15	E. estradiol	20[8]	Barr	W(LG)LBl	c
Lessina	Levonorgestrel	0.1	E. estradiol	20	Barr	P(W)	i
Levlen	Levonorgestrel	0.15	E. estradiol	30	Berlex	O (P)	d
Levlite	Levonorgestrel	0.1	E. estradiol	20	Berlex	P (W)	i
Levora	Levonorgestrel	0.15	E. estradiol	30	Watson	W (Pe)	a
Loestrin 1/20	Nor. acetate	1.0	E. estradiol	20	Parke-Davis	W (Br)[7]	c
Loestrin 1.5/30	Nor. acetate[2]	1.5	E. estradiol	30	Parke-Davis	G (Br)	e
Lo/Ovral	Norgestrel	0.3	E. estradiol	30	Wyeth	W (P)	d
Low-Ogestrel	Norgestrel	0.3	E. estradiol	30	Watson	W (Pe)	a
Microgestin 1/20	Nor. acetate	1.0	E. estradiol	20	Watson	W (Br)[7]	c
Microgestin 1.5/30	Nor. acetate[2]	1.5	E. estradiol	30	Watson	G(Br)[7]	e

(continued)

TABLE 5: COMPOSITION AND IDENTIFICATION OF ORAL CONTRACEPTIVES (Continued)

Name	Progestin	mg/tablet	Estrogen	mcg/tablet	Manufacturer	Color A/IA[5,6]	Inactive Ingredient[9]
Mircette	Desogestrel	0.15	E. estradiol	20[8]	Organon	W (G)(Y)	c
Modicon	Norethindrone	0.5	E. estradiol	35	Ortho	W (G)	f
Necon 0.5/35	Norethindrone	0.5	E. estradiol	35	Watson	LY (W)	a
Necon 1/35	Norethindrone	1.0	E. estradiol	35	Watson	Y (W)	a
Necon 1/50M	Norethindrone	1.0	Mestranol	50	Watson	Bl (W)	a
Nelova 1/50M	Norethindrone	1.0	Mestranol	50	Warner Chilcott	LBl (W)	a
Nordette	Levonorgestrel	0.15	E. estradiol	30	Wyeth	Pe (P)	d
Norethin 1/35	Norethindrone	1.0	E. estradiol	35	Roberts	W (B)	b
Norethin 1/50M	Norethindrone	1.0	Mestranol	50	Roberts	W (B)	b
Norinyl 1/35	Norethindrone	1.0	E. estradiol	35	Watson	G (O)	a
Norinyl 1/50	Norethindrone	1.0	Mestranol	50	Watson	W (O)	a
Norlestrin 1/50	Nor. acetate	1.0	E. estradiol	50	Parke-Davis	Y (W)(Br)[7]	e
Nortrel 0.5/35	Norethindrone	0.5	E. estradiol	35	Barr	LY(W)	f
Nortrel 1/35	Norethindrone	1.0	E. estradiol	35	Barr	Y(W)	f
Ogestrel	Norgestrel	0.5	E. estradiol	50	Watson	W (Pe)	h
Ortho-Cept	Desogestrel	0.15	E. estradiol	30	Ortho	O (G)	c
Ortho-Cyclen	Norgestimate	0.25	E. estradiol	35	Ortho	Bl (G)	f
Ortho-Novum 1/35	Norethindrone	1.0	E. estradiol	35	Ortho	O (G)	f
Ortho-Novum 1/50	Norethindrone	1.0	Mestranol	50	Ortho	Y (G)	f
Ovcon 35	Norethindrone	0.4	E. estradiol	35	Warner Chilcott	Pe (G)	a

108

Ovcon 50	Norethindrone	1.0	E. estradiol	50	Warner Chilcott	Y (G)	g
Ovral	Norgestrel	0.5	E. estradiol	50	Wyeth	W (P)	d
Portia	Levonorgestrel	0.15	E. estradiol	30	Barr	P(W)	h
Sprintec	Norgesimate	0.25	E. estradiol	35	Barr	Bl(W)	h
Yasmin	Drospirenone	3.0	E. estradiol	30	Berlex	Y(W)	i
Zovia 1/35	Ethy. diacetate	1.0	E. estradiol	35	Watson	LP (W)	a
Zovia 1/50	Ethy. diacetate	1.0	E. estradiol	50	Watson	P (W)	a
Extended-Cycle[4]							
Seasonale	Levonorgestrel	0.15	E. estradiol	30	Duramed	P (W)	j
Multiphasic[5]							
Cyclessa	Desogestrel	0.100(7)	E. estrodial	25(7)	Organon	Y	c
	Desogestrel	0.125(7)	E. estrodial	25(7)	Organon	W	c
	Desogestrel	0.150(7)	E. estrodial	25(7)	Organon	O(G)	c
Enpresse	Levonorgestrel	0.05(6)	E. estradiol	30(6)	Barr	P	d
	Levonorgestrel	0.075(5)	E. estradiol	40(5)	Barr	W	d
	Levonorgestrel	0.125(10)	E. estradiol	30(10)	Barr	O(LG)	d

(continued)

109

TABLE 5: COMPOSITION AND IDENTIFICATION OF ORAL CONTRACEPTIVES (*Continued*)

Name	Progestin	mg/tablet	Estrogen	mcg/tablet	Manufacturer	Color A/IA[5,6]	Inactive Ingredient[9]
Estrostep	Nor. acetate	1.0(5)	E. estradiol	20(5)	Warner Chilcott	W,[T]	e
	Nor. acetate	1.0(7)	E. estradiol	30(7)	Warner Chilcott	W,[S]	e
	Nor. acetate	1.0(9)	E. estradiol	35(9)	Warner Chilcott	W,[R] (Br)[8]	e
Necon 10/11	Norethindrone	0.5(10)	E. estradiol	35(10)	Watson	LY	a
	Norethindrone	1.0(11)	E. estradiol	35(11)	Watson	DY	a
Nelova 10/11	Norethindrone	0.5(10)	E. estradiol	35(10)	Warner Chilcott	Y	a
	Norethindrone	1.0(11)	E. estradiol	35(11)	Warner Chilcott	DY (W)	a
Nortrel 7/7/7	Norethindrone	0.5(7)	E. estradiol	35(7)	Barr	LY(W)	f
	Norethindrone	0.75(7)	E. estradiol	35(7)	Barr	Y(W)	f
	Norethindrone	1.0(7)	E. estradiol	35(7)	Barr	Y(W)	f
Ortho-Novum 7/7/7	Norethindrone	0.5(7)	E. estradiol	35(7)	Ortho	W	f
	Norethindrone	0.75(7)	E. estradiol	35(7)	Ortho	LPe	f
	Norethindrone	1.0(7)	E. estradiol	35(7)	Ortho	Pe(G)	f
Ortho-Novum 10/11	Norethindrone	0.5(10)	E. estradiol	35(10)	Ortho	W	f
	Norethindrone	1.0(11)	E. estradiol	35(11)	Ortho	Pe(G)	f
Ortho Tri-Cyclen	Norgestimate	0.180(7)	E. estradiol	35(7)	Ortho	W	f
	Norgestimate	0.215(7)	E. estradiol	35(7)	Ortho	LBl	f
	Norgestimate	0.250(7)	E. estradiol	35(7)	Ortho	Bl(G)	f

Ortho Tri-Cyclen® LO	Norgestimate	0.180(7)	E. estradiol	25(7)	Ortho	W	f
	Norgestimate	0.215(7)	E. estradiol	25(7)	Ortho	LBl	f
	Norgestimate	0.250(7)	E. estradiol	25(7)	Ortho	DBl	f
Tri-Levlen	Levonorgestrel	0.05(6)	E. estradiol	30(6)	Berlex	Br	d
	Levonorgestrel	0.075(5)	E. estradiol	40(5)	Berlex	W	d
	Levonorgestrel	0.125(10)	E. estradiol	30(10)	Berlex	Y(G)	d
Tri-Norinyl	Norethindrone	0.5(7)	E. estradiol	35(7)	Watson	Bl	a
	Norethindrone	1.0(9)	E. estradiol	35(9)	Watson	G	a
	Norethindrone	0.5(5)	E. estradiol	35(5)	Watson	Bl(O)	a
Triphasil	Levonorgestrel	0.05(6)	E. estradiol	30(6)	Wyeth	Br	d
	Levonorgestrel	0.075(5)	E. estradiol	40(5)	Wyeth	W	d
	Levonorgestrel	0.125(10)	E. estradiol	30(10)	Wyeth	Y (G)	d
Trivora	Levonorgestrel	0.05(6)	E.estradiol	30.(6)	Watson	Bl	a
	Levonorcgestrel	0.075(5)	E.estradiol	40(5)	Watson	W	a
	Levonorgestrel	0.125(10)	E.estradiol	30(10)	Watson	P(Pe)	a
Progestin Only							
Camila	Norethindrone	0.35	None	—	Barr	LP	a
Errin	Norethindrone	0.35	None	—	Barr	W(Y)	f
Micronor	Norethindrone	0.35	None	—	Ortho	G	f
Nor-QD	Norethindrone	0.351	None	—	Watson	Y	a
Ovrette	Norgestrel	0.075	None	—	Wyeth	Y	d

(continued)

111

1. Ethynodiol diacetate
2. Norethindrone acetate
3. Ethinylestradiol
4. 91 day regimen, 84 days active tablets
5. Multiphasic product: Number in parenthesis equals days of each phase
6. Color and shape abbreviations are:

Bl-Blue, Br-Brown, DY-Dark
Yellow, G-Green, LG-Light Green,
LPe-Peach, LBl-Light Blue, LP Light
Pink, LY-Light Yellow, O-Orange,
P-Pink, Pe-Peach or Light Orange,
Ro-Rose, W-White,
Y-Yellow, T-Triangular,
S-Square, R-Round.

Color in parenthesis means inactive tablets

7. Inactive brown tablets (Br) contain 75 mg ferrous fumarate
8. E-estadiol(Y) 10mcg for last five days of progestin free interval
9. Inactive Ingredients are listed, below

Symbols for Inactive Ingredients shown in last column of Table 5
Each OC listed in Table 5 contains several Inactive Ingredients (IAs); that "group" is denoted by a letter (e.g. h) in the last column. Below, a table of those group letters shows the number of each particular (IA), and corresponds to a number and IA in the subsequent list. Groups which contain lactose and/or talc are shown in bold, because some patients may be sensitive to lactose; and talc may be carcinogenic.

Inactive Ingredient Groups

a. **21**,24,33,35
b. 3,5,10,17,33
c. 8,10,28,33,37,41
d. 7,**21**,24,30
e. 1,9,**21**,24,26,36,**39**
f. **21**,24,26,34
g. 12,24,33,35
h. 11,**21**,24,26,33
i. 4,10,14,18,**22**,23,24,27,31,33,34,38,**39**,40
j. 2,18,24,32,40
k. 7,16,19,20,**21**,24,30,40,42
l. **22**,24,26,31,34

Inactive Ingredients in a Group

1. Acadia
2. Anhydrous lactose
3. Calcium acetate
4. Calcium carbonate
5. Calcium phosphate
6. Calcium sulphate
7. Cellulose
8. Colloidal silicon dioxide
9. Confectioner's sugar
10. Cornstarch
11. Croscarmellose soldium
12. Dibasic-calcium phosphate
13. Ferric acid
14. Ferric Oxide Pigment
15. Glycerine
16. Glycol
17. Hydrogenated caster oil
18. Hydroxylpropyl methylcellulose
19. Hypro mellose
20. Iron oxide
21. **Lactose**
22. **Lactose monohydrate**
23. Macrogol
24. Magnesium stearate
25. Methylcellulose
26. Microcrystalline cellulose
27. Modified Starch
28. Monohydrate
29. Montanglycol wax
30. Polacrilin potassium
31. Polyethlene glycol
32. Polysorbate 80
33. Povidone
34. Pregelatinized starch
35. Sodium starch glycolate
36. Starch
37. Stearic acid
38. Sucrose
39. **Talc**
40. Titanium dioxide
41. Vitamin E
42. Wax E

TABLE 6: CONTRACEPTIVE PILL ACTIVITY*
[Ranked According to Estrogen Content and Endometrial Potency]

Drug	Endometrial Activity: % Spotting, and bleeding, in third cycle of use[1]	Estrogenic Activity: mcg Ethinyl Estradiol equivalents per day[2]	Progestational Activity: mg Norethindrone equivalents per day[3]	Androgenic Activity: mg Methyl-testosterone per 28 days[4]
50 mcg Estrogen				
Ogestrel/Ovral	4.5	42	1.3	0.80
Necon/Nelova/Norethin/Norinyl/ Ortho-Novum 1/50	10.6	32	1.0	0.34
Ovcon 50	11.9	50	1.0	0.34
Norlestrin 1/50	13.6	39	1.2	0.53
Demulen 50/Zovia 1/50	13.9	26	1.4	0.21
Sub-50 mcg Estrogen				
Monophasic				
Cryselle/Lo-Ovral/Low-Ogestrel	9.6	25	0.8	0.46
Ovcon 35	11.0	40	0.4	0.15
Apri/Desogen/Ortho-Cept	13.1	30	1.5	0.17
Levlen/Levora/Nordette/Portia	14.0	25	0.8	0.46
Ortho-Cyclen/Sprintec	14.3	35	0.4	0.18
Yasmin	14.5	30	1.5	0.00
Necon/Nelova/Norinyl/ Norethin/ Nortrel/Ortho-Novum 1/35	14.7	38	1.0	0.34
Kariva/Mircette	19.7	22	1.5	0.17

Brevicon/Modicon/Necon/ Nortrel .5/35	24.6	42	0.5	0.17
Loestrin/Microgesten 1.5/30	25.2	14	1.7	0.80
Alesse/Aviana/Lessina/Levlite	26.5	17	0.5	0.31
Loestrin 1/20	29.7	13	1.2	0.53
Microgestin 1/20	29.7	13	1.2	0.21
Demulen/Zovia 1/35	37.4	19	1.4	0.21
Seasonale	58.5[5]	316	1.06	0.566
Sub-50 mcg Estrogen				
Multiphasic				
Cyclessa	11.1	25	1.2	0.14
Ortho Tri-Cyclene(r) LO	11.5	25	0.3	0.15
Nortrel 7/7/7/Ortho-Novum 7/7/7	14.5	40	0.8	0.25
Enpresse/Tri-Levlen/Triphasil/Trivora	15.1	28	0.5	0.29
Necon/Nelova/Ortho-Novum 10/11	17.6	40	0.8	0.25
Ortho Tri-Cyclen	17.7	35	0.3	0.15
Estrostep	21.7	16	1.2	0.53
Tri-Norinyl	25.5	40	0.7	0.23
Progestin-Only				
Ovrette	34.9	0	0.20	0.12
Camila/Errin/Micronor/Nor-QD	42.3	1	0.35	0.13

(continued)

115

*The activity of extended cycle regimen is determined by multiplying activity of an ingredient (shown above) for a 21-day cycle by 1.23

1. Information submitted to the United States Food and Drug Administration by the manufacturer. These rates are derived from separate studies conducted by different investigators in several population groups, and therefore, a precise comparison cannot be made, except when randomized comparative studies are used. Randomized comparative studies used are: NDA 18–984 (Ortho 7/7/7 and Jenest vs. Ortho 1 + 35): NDA 19–653 (Ortho-Cyclen vs. Lo/Ovral); Syntex Laboratories study 17–6288 (Tri-Norinyl and Ortho 10/11 vs. Norinyl 1 + 35). Includes bleeding any day that active (progestin-containing) pills are taken.

2. Estrogenic activity of entire tablet - mouse uterine assay. (see Chihal HJW, Dickey RP, Peppler R: Estrogen potency of oral contraceptive pills. Am J Obstet Gynecol 1975;121:75–83, and Dickey RP, Chihal HJW, Peppler R: Potency of three new low-estrogen pills. Am J Obstet Gynecol 1976;125:976–979)

3. Induction of glycogen vacucies in human endometrium (see Dickey RP, Berger GS: Persistent amenorrhea and galactorrhea. In: Clinical Use of Sex Steroids. Givens JR (ed.) Chicago: Yearbook Medical Publishing, 1980;329–38 and Grant EC: Hormone balance of oral contraceptives. J Obstet Gynecol 1967;74:908–918)

4. Rat ventral prostate assay (see Phillips A et al.: Progestational and androgenic receptor binding affinities and in vitro activities of norgestimate and other progestins. Contraception 1990;41:399–410 and Tausk M, de Visser J: International Encyclopedia of Pharmacology and Therapeutics. Ch. 28, Sect. 48, Vol. II. Elmsford, NY: Pergamon Press, 1972)

5. Seasonale. percent reporting any unscheduled BTB or spotting during 2nd 4th 84-day cycle; average 6 days. (see Anderson FD, Hait H. the Seasonale-301 Study Group. A multicenter, randomized study of an extended cycle oral contraceptive. Contraception 2003;68:89–96)

6. Active pills taken for 337 days/year vs. 274 days/year for 28 day regimens; Estrogenic, Progestational, Androgenic activity Multiplied x 1.23.

TABLE 7: EFFECT OF ORAL CONTRACEPTIVES AND COMPONENTS ON SERUM HIGH-DENSITY LIPOPROTEIN CHOLESTEROL (HDL-C) AND LOW-DENSITY LIPOPROTEIN CHOLESTEROL (LDL-C)

						Percent Change From Controls			
					STUDY 5		STUDY 6	
Preparation Progestin mg/Estrogen mcg	STUDY 1*	STUDY 2**	STUDY 3	STUDY 4**	STUDY 5		STUDY 6	
	Hdl-C	Hdl-C	Hdl-C	Hdl-C	Hdl-C	Ldl-C	Hdl-C	Ldl-C
Estrogen-Only								
Ethinyl estradiol 20	+28	+21	—	—	—	—	—	—
Ethinyl estradiol 50	+25	+46						
Progestin-Only								
Levonorgestrel 0.03	—	-2	—	—	—	—	—	—
Medroxyprogesterone acetate 50 IM	-25	-15						
Norethindrone 0.35	—	-4	—	—	—	—	—	—
Norethindrone acetate 1	—	-7	—	—	—	—	—	—
Norethindrone acetate 2	—	-11	—	—	—	—	—	—
Combination OC with Norethindrone								
Ortho-Novum/Norinyl 1/50	0	-8	+1.8	+7.3	-4.1	-5.8	—	—
Ortho-Novum/Norinyl 1/35*	—	-11	—	—	+9.8	-12.1	—	—
Brevicon/Modicon 0.5/35	—	-2	—	—			—	—

(continued)

117

TABLE 7: EFFECT OF ORAL CONTRACEPTIVES AND COMPONENTS ON SERUM HIGH-DENSITY LIPOPROTEIN CHOLESTEROL (HDL-C) AND LOW-DENSITY LIPOPROTEIN CHOLESTEROL (LDL-C) (Cont.)

Preparation Progestin mg/Estrogen mcg	STUDY 1*	STUDY 2**	STUDY 3	STUDY 4**	STUDY 5	STUDY 6
Biphasic OC with Norethindrone						
Necon/Nelova 10/11						
Ortho-Novum 10/11 0.5–1.0/35/	—	—	—	—	+4.6	—
					−6.7	—
Combination OC with Norethindrone Acetate						
Norlestrin 1 1/20	+1	−10	+1.8	−3.6	—	—
Combination OC with Ethynodiol Diacetate						
Demulen 1/35/Zovia 1/35	+10	−13	—	+5.5	—	—
Combination OC with Levonorgestrel or						
dl-Norgestrel						
Ogestrel/Ovral 0.5/30	−16	−12	—	−18.2	−15.6	—
Levlen/Levora/Nordette 0.15/30	—	—	—	—	−4.6	—
					+0.4	—
					+1.2	—
Triphasic OC with Levonorgestrel						
Tri-Levlen/Triphasil/Trivora 0.15–0.25/30	—	—	—	—	+1.2	—
					−3.3	—
Combination OC with Desogestrel						
Desogen/Ortho-Cept 0.15/30	—	—	—	—	+12.1	+12.9
Mircette 0.15/20***	—	—	—	—	−13.8	+15.1
					—	−2.1
						—

Combination OC with Gestodene Not available in the U.S. 0.75/30	—	—	—	—	—	+8.1	−2.5
Combination OC with Norgestimate Ortho-Cyclen 0.25/35	—	—	—	—	—	+7.4	+3.4
Triphasic OC with Norgestimate Ortho Tri-Cyclen 0.18–0.25/35	—	—	—	—	—	+10.5	+2.1

*Length of OC use 21 days
**Length of OC use variable
***NDA information cycle 6

Study 1 in Kloosterboer HJ, Deckers GHJ: Desogestrel: A selective progestogen. Int Proc J 1989;1:26–30
Study 2 in Rooks JB et al.: Epidemiology of hepatocellular adenoma: The role of oral contraceptive use. JAMA 1979;242(7):644–648
Study 3 in World Health Organization (WHO) Scientific Group on Cardiovascular Disease and Steroid Hormone Contraception. Cardiovascular disease and steroid hormone contraception: A report of a WHO scientific group. WHO technical report series 877; 1997;Geneva
Study 4 in Vessey MP, Doll R: Investigation of relation between use of oral contraceptives and thromboembolic disease. Br Med J 1968;2:199–205
Study 5 in Glasier A, Thong KJ, Dewar M et al.: Mifepristone (RU 486) compared with high-dose estrogen and progestogen for emergency post-coital contraception. 1992;327:1041–1044
Study 6 in Sivin I: International experience with Norplant® and Norplant-2® contraceptives. Stud Fam Plann 1988;19:81–94

TABLE 8: CHOICE OF AN INITIAL ORAL CONTRACEPTIVE

After the initial cycles, all patients should be switched to Group 1–10 OCs (< 35 mcg estrogen, low or intermediate androgen activity).

Characteristics	Type of OC Indicated	Suggested OC for the Initial Cycles [See Table 9 for OC Groups]
Regular light menses. 2 to 4 days flow: Mild or no cramps.	Low endometrial activity.	Groups 3, 6, 8
Regular moderate menses. 4 to 6 days flow: Moderate cramps	Intermediate endometrial activity.	Groups 2, 4, 5, 7, 9, 10, 11
Regular heavy menses. 6-plus days flow: Severe cramps.	High endometrial activity.	Group 13
Irregular and infrequent menses, hypermenorrhea when occurs: Associated acne, oily skin, hirsutism.	Probably polycystic ovarian syndrome. High progestational and low androgenic activity desirable.	Groups 2, 6, 7, 8, 10
Irregular menses, hypomenorrhea when occurs: No androgen effects.	If galactorrhea present, possible pituitary adenoma. Skull x-ray or prolactin needed. If no galactorrhea, low estrogen and low progestational activity combination OCs or Multiphasic OCs may be used.	Groups 1, 5, 8, barrier and spermicidal methods
Smokers-Ages 35 and over	Combination OCs contraindicated	Group 1, barrier and spermicidal methods
Nonsmokers-Ages 35 and over	Sub 35 mcg estrogen, intermediate/high progestin, combination OC	20–25 mcg EE OCs from Groups 2, 3, 5, 7, 8

Condition	Recommendation	Groups
Weight less than 110 lbs.	Lower estrogen and low progestin dose	Groups 5, 7, 8 or any Tri-Phasic OC
Weight more than 160 lbs.	High estrogen and intermediate to high progestin dose	Groups 11, 12, 13
Progesterone hypersensitivity: History of toxemia, strong family history of hypertension, excessive weight gain, tiredness or varicose veins during pregnancy, depression, excessive premenstrual edema	Low progestin dose and progestational activity. Monitor blood pressure.	Groups 1, 8, 10 (antimineralocorticoid activity) or any Tri-Phasic
Estrogen hypersensitivity: Excessive nausea, edema or hypertension in pregnancy; hypertrophy of the cervix or uterus; uterine fibroids; large or fibrocystic breasts; heavy menses; migraine.	Low estrogenic activity.	Group 1, or any 20 mcg EE OC
Conditions predisposing to cardiovascular disease, type II hyperlipidemia (hypercholeserolemia), diabetes mellitus, obesity, smoking more than 15 cigarettes per day, hypertension, varicose veins, thrombophlebitis during pregnarcy, family history of cardiovascular disease before age 50	Combination pills not recommended.	Group 1, barrier and spermicidal methods
Surgery planned within one to four weeks.	Combination pills should be stopped	Group 1, barrier and spermicidal methods

TABLE 9: ORAL CONTRACEPTIVES WITH SIMILAR ENDOMETRIAL, PROGESTATIONAL, AND ANDROGENIC ACTIVITIES[1]

Group	Oral Contraceptives	Estrogen And Dose	Activity
#1	Camila, Errin Micronor, Nor-QD Ovrette	No estrogen No estrogen No estrogen	Endometrial: Low Progestational: Low Androgenic: Low
#2	Kariva, Mircette, Apri,Desogen, Ortho-Cept	22 mcg ethinyl estradiol (Average) 30 mcg ethinyl estradiol 30 mcg ethinyl estradiol	Endometrial: Intermediate Progestational: High Androgenic: Low
#3	Loestrin 1/20, Microgestin 1/20 Seasonale, Estrostep* Loestrin 1.5/30, Microgestin 1.5/30	20 mcg ethinyl estradiol 30 mcg ethinyl estradiol 30 mcg ethinyl estradiol	Endometrial: Low Progestational: Intermediate/High Androgenic: Intermediate/High
#4	Cryselle, Levlen, Levora, LoOvral Low-Ogestrel, Nordette Portia	30 mcg ethinyl estradiol 30 mcg ethinyl estradiol 30 mcg ethinyl estradiol	Endometrial: Intermediate Progestational: Intermediate Androgenic: Intermediate
#5	OrthoTri-Cyclen LO* Empresse*,Tri-Levien* Triphasil*, Trivora* Ovcon 35, Ortho-Cyclen Ortho Tri-Cyclen*, Spintec	25 mcg ethinyl estradiol 32 mcg ethinyl estradiol (Average) 32 mcg ethinyl estradiol (Average) 35 mcg ethinyl estradiol 35 mcg ethinyl estradiol	Endometrial: Intermediate Progestational: Low Androgenic: Low
#6	Demulen 1/35 Zovia 1/35	35 mcg ethinyl estradiol	Endometrial: Low Progestational: High Angdrogenic: Low

122

#7	Cyclessa* Necon 10/11*, Nelova 10/11* Ortho-Novum 10/11* Nortrel 7/7/7, Ortho-Novum 7/7/7*	25 mcg ethinyl estradiol 35 mcg ethinyl estradiol 35 mcg ethinyl estradiol 35 mcg ethinyl estradiol	Endometrial: Intermediate Progestational: Intermediate Androgenic: Low
#8	Alesse, Aviane Levlite, Lesinra Brevicon, Modicon Necon 0.5/35, Nelova 0.5/35 Nortrel 0.5/35, Tri-Norinyl*	20 mcg ethinyl estradiol 20 mcg ethinyl estradiol 35 mcg ethinyl estradiol 35 mcg ethinyl estradiol 35 mcg ethinyl estradiol	Endometrial: Low Progestational: Low Androgenic: Low
#9	Necon 1/35, Norethin 1/35 Norinyl 1/35, Nortrel 1/35 Ortho-Novum 1/35	35 mcg ethinyl estradiol 35 mcg ethinyl estradiol 35 mcg ethinyl estradiol	Endometrial: Intermediate Progestational: Intermediate Androgenic: Intermediate
#10	Yasmin	30 mcg ethinyl estradiol	Endometrial: Intermediate Progestational: High Androgenic: none (Anti-androgenic)**
#11	Demulen 1/50 Zovia 1/50	50 mcg ethinyl estradiol	Endometrial: Intermediate Progestational: High Androgenic: Low
#12	Necon 1/50M, Norethin 1/50M Norinyl 1/50, Nelova 1/50M Ortho-Novum 1/50 Norlestrin 1/50, Ovcon 1/50	50 mcg mestranol 50 mcg mestranol 50 mcg mestranol 50 mcg ethinyl estradiol	Endometrial: Intermediate Progestational: Intermediate Androgenic: Intermediate
#13	Ogestrel Ovral	50 mcg ethinyl estradiol	Endometrial: High Progestational: High Androgenic: High

1. Arranged by estrogen type and dose; see Table 6 for specific activity.
* Multiphasic
** Antimineralocorticoid activity

TABLE 10: LABORATORY CHANGES ASSOCIATED WITH ORAL CONTRACEPTIVE USE

ESTROGEN RELATED		PROGESTIN-RELATED
SERUM INCREASED	**SERUM INCREASED**	**SERUM INCREASED**
Aldosterone	Prolactin	Fibrinolysis
Amylase	Prothrombin time	Hematocrit
Ceruloplasmin	Renin substrate	Insulin
Clotting factors II, VII, VIII, IX, X, XI and prothrombin	(angiotensinogen and renin)	Insulin resistance
Cortisol	Sex steroid binding globulin (testosterone)	Nitrogen
Erythrocyte sedimentation rate	Sodium	Ratio total cholesterol and/or HDL-cholesterol/LDL-cholesterol
Fibrinogen	T4 thyroxine	
Free fatty acids	Thyroxine binding globulin	
FSH	Total lipids	**SERUM DECREASED**
Growth hormone	Transferrin	Alpha amino nitrogen
HDL-cholesterol	Triglycerides	Complement reactive protein
LDL-cholesterol		HDL-cholesterol
Protein-bound iodine	**SERUM DECREASED**	Luteinizing hormone
Platelet count, aggregation and cohesiveness	Albumin	Triglycerides
Plasmin	Antithrombin III	
Plasminogen	Glucose absorption	
	Insulin	
	Prothrombin time	
	Ratio total cholesterol/HDL cholesterol	
	Triiodothyronine resin uptake (T3)	
	SERUM ALTERED	
	ACTH response	
	Bromsulphalein test	
	Glucose tolerance test	
	Lupus erythematosus cell prep	
	Metapyrone test	
	URINE INCREASED	
	Aldosterone	
	URINE DECREASED	
	Gonadotropins	

124

ETIOLOGY UNKNOWN

SERUM INCREASED	SERUM INCREASED	SERUM DECREASED	URINE INCREASED
Alkaline phosphatase	Iron	Ascorbic acid	Coproporphyrin
Alpha 1 antitrypsin	Iron binding capacity	Calcium	Delta-aminolevulinic acid
Alpha 1, alpha 2 globulin	Lactate	Cholinesterase	Formiminoglutamic acid
Angiotensin I and II	Leukocyte	Erythrocyte count	excretion after histidine
Antinuclear antibodies	Lipoproteins alpha, beta,	Folate	Porphyrins
Bilirubin	pre-beta, total	Haptoglobin	Xanthurenic acid
Cephalin flocculation	Nucleotidase	Magnesium	
Copper	(5-nucleotidase)	Renin	*URINE DECREASED*
Cryofibrinogen	PPT	Vitamin B_{12}	17-hydroxy steroids
Erythrocyte sedimentation rate	Phospholipids	Zinc	17-keto steroids
Euglobulin lysis	Plasma volume		Calcium
Formiminoglutamic acid	Pyruvate		Estrogen (-diol, -triol)
excretion after histidine	SGOT		Etiocholanolone
Gamma glutamyl/	SGPT		Pregnanediol, (-triol)
transpeptidase	Sodium		Tetrahydrocannabinol
Immunoglobulin A	Transaminase		Urobilinogen
Immunoglobulin G	Vitamin A		
Immunoglobulin M			

125

TABLE 11: SIDE EFFECTS RELATED TO HORMONE CONTENT

I. REPRODUCTIVE SYSTEM	II. PREMENSTRUAL SYNDROME
ESTROGEN EXCESS Breast cystic changes Cervical extrophy Dysmenorrhea Hypermenorrhea, menorrhagia, and clotting Increase in breast size Mucorrhea Uterine enlargement Uterine fibroid growth *ESTROGEN DEFICIENCY* Absence of withdrawal bleeding Bleeding and spotting during pill days 1 to 9 Continuous bleeding and spotting Flow decrease, hypomenorrhea Pelvic relaxation symptoms Vaginitis atrophic	*PROGESTIN EXCESS* Cervicitis Flow length decrease Moniliasis *PROGESTIN DEFICIENCY* Breakthrough bleeding and spotting during pill days 10 to 21 Delayed withdrawal bleeding Dysmenorrhea (also estrogen excess) Heavy flow and clots (also estrogen excess), hypermenorrhea, menorrhagia	*ESTROGEN EXCESS OR PROGESTERONE DEFICIENCY* Bloating Dizziness, syncope Edema Headache (cyclic) Irritability Leg cramps Nausea, vomiting Visual changes (cyclic) Weight gain (cyclic)

III. GENERAL		IV. CARDIOVASCULAR SYSTEM
ESTROGEN EXCESS Chloasma Chronic nasal pharyngitis Gastric influenza and varicella Hay fever and allergic rhinitis Urinary tract infection *ESTROGEN DEFICIENCY* Nervousness Vasomotor symptoms	*PROGESTIN EXCESS* Appetite increase Depression Fatigue Hypoglycemia symptoms Libido decrease *ANDROGEN EXCESS* Acne Cholestatic jaundice Hirsutism Libido increase Oily skin and scalp Rash and pruritus Edema	*PROGESTIN EXCESS* Hypertension Leg vein dilation *ESTROGEN EXCESS* Capillary fragility Cerebrovascular accident Deep vein thrombosis hemiparesis (unilateral weakness and numbness) Telangiectasias Thromboembolic disease

TABLE 12: SYMPTOMS OF A SERIOUS OR POTENTIALLY SERIOUS NATURE

SYMPTOM	POSSIBLE CAUSE
SERIOUS: Pills should be stopped immediately.	
Loss of vision, proptosis, diplopia, papilledema	Retinal artery thrombosis
Unilateral numbness, weakness or tingling	Hemorrhagic or thrombotic stroke
Severe pains in chest, left arm or neck	Myocardial infarction
Hemoptysis	Pulmonary embolism
Severe pains, tenderness or swelling, warmth or palpable cord in legs	Thrombophlebitis
Slurring of speech	Hemorrhagic or thrombotic stroke
Hepatic mass or tenderness	Liver neoplasm

POTENTIALLY SERIOUS: Pills may be continued with caution while patient is being evaluated	
Absense of menses	Pregnancy
Spotting or breakthrough bleeding	Cervical endomentrial or vaginal cancer
Breast mass, pain or swelling	Breast cancer
Right upper-quadrant pain	Cholecystitis, cholelithiasis or liver neoplasm
Mid-epigastric pain	Thrombosis of abdominal artery or vein, myocardial Infarction or pulmonary embolism
Migraine (vascular or throbbing) headache	Vascular spasm which may precede thrombosis
Severe nonvascular headache	Hypertension, vascular spasm
Galactorrhea	Pituitary adenoma
Jaundice, pruitus	Cholestatic jaundice
Depression, sleepiness	B_6 deficiency
Uterine size increase	Leiomyomata, adenomyosis, pregnancy

TABLE 13: VITAMIN AND MINERAL CHANGES ASSOCIATED WITH ORAL CONTRACEPTIVES

NUTRIENT	SERUM PLASMA OR BLOOD LEVEL CHANGES	EARLY CLINICAL EFFECTS	MINIMUM DAILY REQUIREMENTS ADULTS	BEST DIETARY SOURCES
Vitamin A	Increased	Fissured skin, coarsening of hair, hepatomegaly	4,000 to 5,000 IU	Liver, kidney, dairy products, eggs
Thiamine (B_1)	Decreased	Anorexia, lethargy, depression, irritability (beriberi)	1 mg	Pork, wheat germ
Riboflavin (B_2)	Decreased	Glossitis, seborrhea, fissures of the corners of the mouth, conjunctival irritation	1.2 mg	Milk, cheese
Pyridoxine (B_6)	Decreased	Clinical depression, glucose intolerance	2.0 mg	Yeast, wheat germ, meat, bananas
Cobalamin (B_{12})	Decreased	Potentiates pernicious anemia, folacin deficiency	3 mcg	Liver, kidney, fresh milk

Ascorbic acid (C)	Decreased	Bleeding gums, swollen, tender joints (scurvy)	45 mg	Citrus fruits, raw vegetables, tomatoes
Folacin (folic acid)	Decreased	Megaloblastic anemia gastrointestinal disturbances	0.4 mg	Liver, kidney beans, lima beans, green leafy vegetables
Calcium	Decreased	None	1 gm	Milk, cheese
Copper	Increased	Pigment changes, Wilson's disease (hepatolenticular degeneration)	2 mg	Liver, shellfish, whole grains, cherries
Iron	Increased	None	10 mg	Liver, meat, egg yolk, green leafy vegetables
Magnesium	Decreased	Weight loss, change in hair, depression, muscle weakness	350 mg	Whole grain cereals, nuts, meats, milk
Zinc	Decreased	Delayed wound healing, alopecia, loss of taste	15 mg	Meat, liver, eggs, seafood

Source: Amatayakul K, Uttaravachai C, Singkamani R, Ruckphaopunt S: Vitamin metabolism and the effects of multivitamin supplementation in oral contraceptive users. Contraception 1984; 30(2):179–196

TABLE 14: DRUGS THAT MAY AFFECT ORAL CONTRACEPTIVE ACTIVITIES

CLASS OF COMPOUND	DRUG	PROPOSED METHOD OF ACTION	SUGGESTED MANAGEMENT	REF.
Drugs That May Decrease Oral Contraceptive Steroid Activities				

Anticonvulsant Drugs	Carbamazepine
	Barbiturates:
	  Phenobarbital
	  Primidone
	Hydantoins:
	  Ethotoin
	  Mephenytoin
	  Phenytoin
	Succinimide:
	  Ethosuximide
		Induction of liver microsomal enzymes; rapid metabolism of estrogen and increased binding of progestin and ethinyl estradiol to sex hormone binding globulin.	Use another method, another drug or higher dose OC (50 mcg ethinylestradiol)	1
				2
				3
				4

Cholesterol Lowering Agent	Clofibrate	Reduces elevated serum triglycerides and cholesterol	Use another method	5, 6, 7, 8
Antituberculosis Antibiotics and Antifungals	Ampicillin Cotrimoxazole Griseofulvin Minocycline Penicillin Rifampin	Rifampin increases metabolism of progestins Enterohepatic circulation disturbance, intestinal hurry	For short course, use additional method or use another drug	9 10 11 12

Antituberculosis Antibiotics and Antifungals	Chloramphenicol Metronidazole Neomycin Nitrofurantoin Sulfonamide Tetracycline	Induction of microsomal liver enzymes: see above	For long course, use another method	3 12 13
Sedatives and Hypnotics	Antimigraine preparations Benzodiazepines Chloral hydrate Diazepam	Increased microsomal liver enzymes: see above	For short course, use additional method or another drug For long course, use another method or higher dose OCs	3 14

Drugs That May Increase Oral Contraceptive Steroid Activities

Antipyretics	Acetaminophen Paracetamol	Reduces sulphation of ethinyl estradiol in the gut	None needed unless symptoms of excess estrogen occur	11, 15, 16
Antifungals	Flucorazole	Inhibition of cytochrome P450 oxidation	None needed unless symptoms of excess estrogen occur	17
Other	Ascorbic acid	Inhibition of cytochrome P450 oxidation	None needed unless symptoms of excess estrogen occur	18

References for Table 14: Drugs that may Affect Oral Contraceptive Activities

1. Back DJ et al.: The interaction of phenobarbital and other anticonvulsants with oral contraceptive steroid therapy. Contraception 1980;22(5): 495–503.
2. Coulam CB, Annegers JF: Do anticonvulsants reduce the efficacy of oral contraceptives? Epilepsia 1979;20(5):519–525.
3. Medical Letter. 1981;23:5(578):17–28.
4. Obstetrician's and Gynecologist's Compendium of Drug Therapy. New York: Biomedical Information Corporation, 1981–1982;22:7.
5. Physician's Desk Reference, 35th ed. Oradell, NJ: Medical Economics Company, 1981;606.
6. Back DJ et al.: The effect of rifampicin on norethisterone pharmacokinetics. Eur J Clin Pharmacol 1971;15(3):193–197.
7. Back DJ et al.: Interindividual variation and drug interactions with hormonal steroid contraceptives. Drugs 1981;21(1):46–61.
8. Friedman CI et al.: The effect of ampicillin on oral contraceptive effectiveness. Am J Obstet Gynecol 1980;55(1):33–37.
9. Grimmer SFM, Allen WL, Back DJ, Breckenridge AM, Orme M, et al.: The effect of cotrimoxazole on oral contraceptive steroids in women. Contraception 1983;28:53–59.
10. Joshi JV et al.: A study of interaction of a low-dose combination oral contraceptive with antitubercular drugs. Contraception 1980;21(6):617–629.

11. Shenfield GM, Griffin JM: Clinical pharmacokinetics of contraceptive steroids. Clinical Pharmacokinetic 1991;(I)20:15–37.

12. Dickinson B, Altman RD, Nielsen NH, Sterling ML. Drug interactions between oral contraceptives and antibiotics. Obstet Gynecol 2001;98:853–60.

13. Joshi JV et al.: A study of interaction of a low-dose combination oral contraceptive with ampicillin and metronidazole. Contraception 1980;22(6):643–652.

14. Abernethy DR, Greenb;att DJ, Divoll M, Arendt RL: Impairment of diazepam clearance with low-dose oral contraceptive steroid therapy. Clin Pharmacol Ther 1984;35:360–366.

15. Mitchell MC, Hanew T, Meredith CG, Schenker S: Effects of oral contraceptive steroids on acetaminophen metabolism and elimination. Clin Pharm Ther 1983;34:41–53.

16. Rogers SM, Back, Stevenson PJ, Grimmer SFM, Orme ML: Paracetamol interaction with oral contraceptive steroids: Increased plasma concentrations of ethinyl oestradiol. Br J Clin Pharm 1987;23:721–725.

17. Hilbert J, Messig M, Kuye O, Friedman H. Evaluation of interaction between fluconazole and an oral contraceptive in healthy women. Obstet Gynecol 2001;98:218–23.

18. Back DJ, Orme ML'E. Pharmacokinetic drug interactions with oral contraceptives. Clin Pharmacokinet 1990;18:472–84.

135

TABLE 15: MODIFICATION OF OTHER DRUG ACTIVITY BY ORAL CONTRACEPTIVES

CLASS OF COMPOUND	DRUG	MODIFICATION OF DRUG ACTION	SUGGESTED MANAGEMENT	REF.
Antibiotics	Cyclosporine Troleandomycin	Increased serum levels and possible liver damage	Do not use OC with these antibiotics	1 2
Anticoagulants	All	OCs increase clotting factors, decrease efficacy	Do not use OC with anticoagulant	3 4
Anticonvulsants	All	Fluid retention, increases seizures	Use another method	5, 6, 7, 8
Antidiabetic Agents	Insulin and oral hypoglycemic Agents	High dose OCs cause impaired glucose tolerance	Use low dose estrogen and progestin OC or use another method	4, 9
Antihypertensive Agents	Guanethidine Methyldopa	Estrogen component causes Naretention; progestin has no effect	Use low estrogen OC or another method. Possible need for dosage increase.	4, 10

			11, 12, 13
Alpha-II Adrenoreceptor Agents	Clonidine		
Antipyretics and Analgesics	Acetaminophen Aspirin Morphine	Increased renal clearance	Increased dosage may be necessary	2, 14
	Antipyrine Meperidine	Impaired metabolism	Decrease dosage	15
Benzodiazepines	Alprazolam Bronazepam Chlordiazepoxide Clotiazepam Diazepam Lorazepam Nitrazepam Oxazepam Temazepam Triazolam	Increases effects, decreases clearance or increased metabolism	Use with caution	2 4 16 17
Beta-blocking Agents	Metoprolol Oxprenolol Propanolol	Increases drug effect	Decrease dosage if necessary	2, 4, 18, 19

(continued)

137

TABLE 15: MODIFICATION OF OTHER DRUG ACTIVITY BY ORAL CONTRACEPTIVES (*Continued*)

Class Of Compound	Drug	Modification of Drug Action	Suggested Management	Ref
Betamimetics	Isoproterenol agents	Estrogen causes decreased response to these drugs	Adjust dose of drug as necessary. Discontinuing OCs can result in excessive drug activity	18 20
Bronchodilators	All	Decreases oxidation, leading to Possible toxicity	Use with caution	21
Cholesterol-lowering Agents	Clofibrate	Increased clearance rate	Increase dose	2
Corticosteroids	Prednisone Prednisolone	Markedly increases serum levels	Possible need for dosage decreases	2, 21, 22
Dopamine Agonists	Apomorphine	Decreased effect	Higher doses may be necessary	2, 13
Methylxanthines	Caffeine Theophylline Methylxanthine	Higher serum levels due to decreased clearance	Use with caution	2
Phenothiazine Tranquilizers	All phenothiazines, reserpine, and similar drugs	Estrogen potentiates the hyperprolactinemia effect of these drugs	Use other drugs or lower dose OCs. If galactorrhea or hyperprolactinemia occurs, use other method	23
Tricyclic Antidepressants	Clomipramine Imipramine Amitriptyline	Increased serum levels due to decreased clearance	Decrease dosage or use another method	2, 8, 24

138

References for Table 15: Modification of Other Drug Activity by Oral Contraceptives

1. Friedman CI et al.: The effect of ampicillin on oral contraceptive effectiveness. Am J Obstet Gynecol 1980;55(1):33–37.
2. Shenfield GM, Griffin JM: Clinical pharmacokinetics of contraceptive steroids. Clinical Pharmacokinetic 1991;(I)20:15–37.
3. Beller FK et al.: Effects of oral contraceptives on blood coagulation: A review. Obstet Gynecol Surv 1985;40(7):425–436.
4. Medical Letter. 1981;23:5(578):17–28.
5. Back DJ et al.: The interaction of phenobarbital and other anticonvulsants with oral contraceptive steroid therapy. Contraception 1980;22(5): 495–503.
6. Back J, Grimmer SFM, Orme MLE, Prcudlove C, Mann RD, et al.: Evaluation of Committee on Safety of Medicines yellow card reports on oral contraceptive drug interactions with anticonvulsants and antibiotics. Br J Clin Pharm 1988;25:527–532.
7. Coulam CB, Annegers JF: Do anticonvulsants reduce the efficacy of oral contraceptives? Epilepsia 1979;20(5):519–525.
8. Gringras M, Beaumont G, Grieve A: Clomipramine and oral contraceptives: An interaction study: Clinical findings. J Int Med Res 1980;3:76–80.
9. Szabo AG, Cole HS, Grimaldi RD: Glucose tolerance in gestational diabetic women during and after treatment with the combination type oral contraceptives. N Engl J Med 1970;282:646.
10. Wambach G et al.: Interaction of synthetic progestogens with renal mineral-corticoid receptors. Acta Endocrinol 1979;92(3):560–567.
11. Baciewicz AM: Oral contraceptive drug interactions. Ther Drug Monit 1985;7(1):26–35.
12. Blumenstein BA, Douglas MB, Hall WD: Blood pressure changes and oral contraceptive use: A study of 2,676 black women in the southeastern United States. Am J Epidemiol 1980;112:539–552.

139

13. Chalmers JS, Fulli-Lemaire I, Cowen PJ: Effects of the contraceptive pill on sedative responses to clonidine and apomorphine in normal women. Psych Med 1985;15:363–367.

14. Watson KJR, Ghabrial H, Mashford ML, Harman PJ, Breen KJ, et al.: Effects of sex and the oral contraceptive pill on morphine disposition. Clin Exper Pharmacol Physiol 1987;14:33.

15. Kay CR: Oral contraceptives and cancer. Lancet 1983;2:1018–1021.

16. Ochs HR, Greenblatt DJ, Friedman H, Burstein ES, Locniskz BS, et al.: Bromazepam pharmacokinetics: Influence of age, gender, oral contraceptives, cimetidine, and propranolol. Clin Pharm Ther 1987;41:562–570.

17. Ochs HR, Greenblatt DJ, Verburg-Ochs B, Harmatz JS, Grehl H: Disposition of clotiazepam: Influence of age, sex, oral contraceptives, crimetidine, isoniazid, and ethanol. Europ J Clin Pharm 1984;26:55–59.

18. Fregly MJ, Thrasher TN: Response of heart rate to acute administration of isoproterenol in rats treated chronically with norethynodrel, EE, and both combined. Endocrinology 1977;100(1):148–154.

19. Kendall MJ, Jack DB, Quarterman CP, Smith SR, Zaman R: ß-andrenoceptor blocker pharmacokinetics and the oral contraceptive pill. Br J Clin Phar 1984;17:87S–89S.

20. Federal Drug Administration Drug Bulletin. April 1990;5.

21. Vessey MP, McPherson K, Yeates D: Mortality in oral contraceptive users. Lancet 1981;1:549.

22. Legler UF: Lack of impairment of fluocortolone disposition in oral contraceptive users. Europ J Clin Pharm 1988;35:101–103.

23. Dickey RP, Stone SC: Drugs that affect the breast and lactation. Clin Obstet Gynecol 1975;18:2.

24. Edelbroek PM, Zitman FG, Knoppert-van er Klein EAM, van Putten PM, de Wolff FA: Therapeutic drug monitoring of amitryptiline: Impact of age, smoking, and contraceptives on drug and metabolite levels in bulemic women. Clin Chemica Acta 1987;165:177–187.

140

TABLE 16: CARDIOVASCULAR DISEASE MORTALITY IN ORAL CONTRACEPTIVE USERS AND FORMER USERS, AND CONTROLS

MORTALITY RATE PER 100,000 WOMEN-YEARS

CAUSE	CURRENT USERS	FORMER USERS	CONTROLS	CURRENT USERS VS. CONTROLS	FORMER USERS VS. CONTROLS
All nonrheumatic heart disease and hypertension	15.1	9.6	2.1	7.3	4.6
Ischemic heart disease	13.0	4.1	2.0	6.4	2.0
Malignant hypertension	0.0	2.5	0.0	—	—
All cerebrovascular disease	10.1	18.2	5.0	2.0	3.6
Subarachnoid hemorrhage	7.3	10.2	2.3	3.2	4.5
Cerebral thrombosis, hemorrhage and embolism	2.7	8.1	2.7	1.0	3.0
Pulmonary embolism and thrombophlebitis	2.8	2.2	0.0	—	—
Other vascular diseases	0.8	0.9	0.0	—	—
All circulatory diseases	28.6	30.9	7.2	4.0	4.3

Source: Rosner D, Lane WW: Oral contraceptive use has no adverse effect on the prognosis of breast cancer. Cancer 1986;57(3):591–596.

TABLE 17: INCIDENCE OF AND MORTALITY FROM CARDIOVASCULAR DISEASE (CVD) BY CONDITION, AGE, AND CURRENT OC USE

RATES PER 100,000 WOMEN PER YEAR

INCIDENCE	None	OC Use Old*	OC Use New*
Ages 20 to 24			
Myocardial infarction	0.2	0.5	0.2
Ischemic stroke	1.0	2.5	2.5
Hemorrhagic stroke	2.0	2.0	2.0
Venous thromboembolism	3.0	9.6	7.7 to 21.1
Total CVD (range†)	6.2	14.6	11.4 to 25.8
Ages 40 to 44			
Myocardial infarction	30.0	78.0	30.0
Ischemic stroke	2.0	5.0	5.0
Hemorrhagic stroke	7.0	14.0	14.0
Venous thromboembolism	6.0	19.2	15.4 to 42.2
Total CVD (range†)	45.0	127.0	64.4 to 91.2

142

MORTALITY	OC Use		
Ages 15 to 24	None	Old*	New*
Myocardial infarction	0.1	0.3	0.1
Stroke (all)	1.0	1.5	1.5
Venous thromboembolism	0.1	0.3	0.2 to 0.7
Total CVD mortality (range†)	1.2	2.1	1.8 to 2.3/20

	OC Use		
Ages 35 to 44	None	Old*	New*
Myocardial infarction	3.0	7.8	3.0
Stroke (all)	6.0	12.0	12.0
Venous thromboembolism	0.2	0.6	0.5 to 2.8
Total CVD mortality (range†)	9.2	20.4	15.5 to 17.8

*All OCs containing 50 μg of estrogen or less; most contained 35 μg or less. "Old" refers to OCs containing levonorgestrel or sometimes norethindrone. "New" refers to OCs containing desogestrel or gestodene.

†The range is derived from the published low and high relative risks for the association of each condition with use of OCs.

Adapted from Consensus Conference on Oral Contraceptives and Cardiovascular Disease. Fertil Steril 1999;71(6)Suppl 3.

145

SECTION 19: PATIENT COMPLAINTS CROSS REFERENCE

The following list contains common patient complaints that may be due to side effects occurring because of OC use (also see Tables 11 and 12). Many OC users experience no side effects, and many health problems have no relation to OC use. However, since these symptoms could possibly be caused or aggravated by OC use, they are included in this listing, followed by the section number(s) where information concerning this symptom can be found:

NOTES

SECTION 20: BREAKTHROUGH BLEEDING AND SPOTTING

Clinical Information

Bleeding that requires use of a perineal pad or vaginal tampon during the time active OCs are taken is referred to as breakthrough bleeding (BTB). A lesser amount of bleeding during this period is defined as spotting. Menstrual irregularities such as these are the most common reasons women give for discontinuing OC use while still needing contraception (1).

BTB is most common with low-dose combination OCs and progestin-only pills. It is the most frequent medical reason that women discontinue OC use. It occurs most often during the first cycles of OC use while the endometrium is adjusting to a lower amount of estrogen and progestin than was present during normal menstrual cycle prior to OC use (2, 3, 4).

One-third to one-half of all women who bleed during the first cycle of OC use will not bleed in the second. Bleeding continues to decrease until it reaches a plateau in the second to fourth cycle. The plateau is reached earlier when OCs with higher progestational and androgenic activities are used.

Bleeding that starts early in the cycle (before the tenth OC is taken) or that is mild and continues from the previous cycle is usually due to insufficient estrogen activity. Estrogen-insufficiency bleeding is also associated with failure to menstruate during the seven tablet-free or placebo days of the cycle.

Bleeding that starts after the tenth OC is taken is usually due to insufficient potency or dose of the progestin component. Heavy menses and menstrual cramps may accompany this type of bleeding.

Bleeding and spotting are more common in overweight women (5, 6).

Bleeding and spotting may appear to occur more frequently in extended use cycles. Fifty-eight percent of women reported an episode of BTB or spotting during the second through fourth 84 days of active tablet use in Seasonale® cycles (7). The average duration of bleeding was short 1.8 days.

Causal Factors

BTB and spotting are due to the failure of the synthetic sex hormones in the OC either to provide adequate stimulus to the endometrium and its vessels following menstruation or to maintain the endometrium and vessels until the end of the active OC cycle. This may be due to:

- Inadequate amounts of estrogen and progestin in the OC
- Imbalance between estrogen and progestin components
- Insensitivity of the endometrium to the OC.

Bleeding may also be the result of:
- Missed pills
- Drug interactions
- Endometrial infection (endometritis) (8)
- Adenomyosis.

BTB is 30% more frequent in women who smoke during early pill cycles and increases to 84% more frequent in smokers in the sixth cycle (9). BTB can occur after many months of OC use. Bleeding that begins after OCs have been used for six months or longer may be due to:

- Progressive atrophy of the endometrium
- An increased rate of metabolism of OC steroids
- End organ insensitivity or resistance (tachyphylaxis)
- Drug interactions
- Infection
- Missed pills.

Management

Small amounts of BTB or spotting are not harmful as long as the diet is adequate and the patient accepts the inconvenience. Since bleeding may denote a lack of complete OC efficacy, it is important that clinicians advise patients to use additional contraception until bleeding has completely ceased.

Bleeding may be a result of spontaneous abortion or tubal pregnancy in women who become pregnant while taking OCs. Additionally, bleeding as well as pain may indicate pelvic inflammatory disease (PID) or endometriosis. Thus, the possibility of pregnancy and/or pathological conditions must be eliminated by appropriate examination before a change in OCs is considered.

Bleeding due to inadequate endometrial support can be treated by switching the patient to an OC with greater endometrial activity (see Table 6). Increased endometrial activity may be achieved with:

- Higher progestin doses
- More androgenic progestins
- Multiphasic OCs
- Higher estrogen doses
- Different ratios of estrogen-to-progestin
- Switching to 28 day instead of extended cycle OC.

Switching a patient to an OC with a higher progestational activity is indicated if bleeding begins after day 14 of active OCs (also called early withdrawal bleeding).

Switching a patient to an OC with higher androgenic activity will usually decrease bleeding that begins at any time during the menstrual cycle.

Switching a patient to an OC with a higher estrogen activity is effective only if:

- Bleeding begins during the first 14 days of the cycle
- Menses continues into the active pill cycle
- Absence of withdrawal menses.

The ability of a particular OC to prevent bleeding and spotting is dependent upon the:

- Type of progestin used
- Doses of estrogen and progestin
- Ratio of estrogen-to-progestin.

The column "Endometrial Activity" in Table 6 lists the percentage of women who experience BTB or spotting during the third cycle of OC use. These rates are based on data provided by OC manufacturers to the FDA for newer products and on information published in medical journals for earlier products.

Doses of estrogen greater than 50 mcg are not needed in order to achieve the lowest possible levels of BTB and spotting. Because of the potential long-term adverse effects of progestins and androgens on the vascular system, OCs with low progestational and androgenic potencies as well as low estrogen doses should be chosen over other OCs with similar profiles of bleeding and spotting.

If bleeding continues after an appropriate switch in OCs, a patient should be re-examined for other conditions that may cause bleeding.

New OC patients should be instructed that BTB and spotting may be expected during the first two to four cycles of use. Women can minimize BTB by taking their pills at the same time each day.

References for Section 20: Breakthrough Bleeding and Spotting

1. Pye RJ et al.: Effect of oral contraceptives on sebum excretion rate. Br Med J 1977;2:1581–1582.
2. Dickey RP: Diagnosis and management of patients with oral contraceptive side effects. J Cont Educ Obstet Gynecol 1978;20:19.
3. Dickey RP: The pill: Physiology, pharmacology, and clinical use. In: Seminar in Family Planning, 1st ed. Isenman AW, Knox EG, Tyrer L (eds.) American College of Obstetrics and Gynecology, 1972. 2nd ed., 1974.
4. Dickey RP, Chihal HJW, Peppler R: Potency of three new low-estrogen pills. Am J Obstet Gynecol 1976;125:976–979.
5. Talwar PP, Berger GS: Side effects of drugs: The relation of body weight to side effects associated with oral contraceptives. Br Med J 1977;1:1637–1638.
6. Holt VL, Cushing-Haugen KL, Daling JR. Body weight and risk of oral contraceptive failure. Obstet Gynecol 2002;99:820–7.

7. Anderson FD, Hait H. the Seasonale-301 Study Group. A multi-center randomized study of an extended cycle oral contraceptive. Contraception 2003;68:89–96.

8. Krettek JE, Arkin SI et al.: Chlamydia trachomatis in patients who used oral contraceptives and had intermenstrual spotting. Obstet and Gynecol 1993;81:728–731.

9. Rosenberg MJ, Waugh MS, Stevens CM: Smoking and cycle control among oral contraceptive users. Am J Obstet Gynceol 1996;174:628–632.

NOTES

SECTION 21: HEAVY MENSES/DYSMENORRHEA

HEAVY MENSES

Clinical Information

Heavy menses, also termed hypermenorrhea or menorrhagia, is much less common than decreased flow in OC users. If heavy menses occurs, however, it may be due to progestational deficiency and is sometimes associated with premenstrual bleeding or spotting.

Occasionally, heavy menses may be due to pathological causes, such as:

- Neoplasia of the uterus
- Uterine leiomyoma
- Adenomyosis
- Abnormal pregnancy
- Endometrial polyps.

Causal Factors

Excessively heavy menses, with or without clots, or prolonged menses in OC users may be associated with an insufficient progestational or excessive estrogenic effect. These symptoms are similar to those of nonusers who have anovulatory cycles. A delay in onset of menses until nearly time to restart active OCs is also due to progestational deficiency.

Management

Pathological causes must be ruled out by appropriate methods. To control non-pathological hypermenorrhea, patients may be switched to OCs with greater progestational and androgenic activities and/or lower estrogen doses.

DYSMENORRHEA

Clinical Information

Patients who experienced dysmenorrhea (painful menstruation) prior to OC use often note relief while taking OCs,

156

but women who were anovulatory prior to taking OCs may begin to experience menstrual cramps for the first time.

Dysmenorrhea due to adenomyosis and endometriosis is decreased in OC users, especially when low-estrogen and high progestational-activity OCs are used.

Pain due to uterine descensus may be suspected if pain worsens when patients stand for prolonged periods or lift heavy objects.

Pelvic infection may occur at any time during OC use and it is often accompanied by:
- Breakthrough bleeding or spotting
- Increased or prolonged bleeding during menses
- Dyspareunia.

Causal Factors

The etiology of primary dysmenorrhea is unknown. Proposed causes (1) are:
- Hypercontractility of the uterus due to release of endometrial toxins or prostaglandins
- Vasoconstriction
- Pathological changes within the sacral nerve
- Adenomyosis and endometriosis
- Endometritis and severe cervicitis.

Management

If no pathological conditions are found, menstrual cramps that first occur after starting OCs may be reduced by switching patients to OCs with greater progestational and androgenic activities and less estrogenic activities. However, if symptoms are due to uterine descensus, pain may worsen. If pain is due to uterine descensus, switching patients to OCs with higher estrogen activities may relieve symptoms.

References for Section 21: Heavy Menses/Dysmenorrhea

1. Ramcharan S, Pellegrin FA, Ray RM, Hsu JP: The Walnut Creek Contraceptive Drug Study: A prospective study of the side effects of oral contraceptives. J Reprod Med 1980;25:345–372.

SECTION 22: AMENORRHEA

AMENORRHEA (MISSED MENSES)

Clinical Information

Absence of withdrawal menses during the seven days between active OCs is referred to as silent or missed menses.

Absence of withdrawal menstruation is more common in women taking low estrogen dose OCs that have relatively weak androgenic and progestational activities. Symptoms may first appear after OCs have been taken for several months because a tolerance to estrogen has developed.

Absence of menstruation may be accompanied by breakthrough bleeding (BTB) or spotting during the 21 days in which active OCs are taken.

Absence of menses may also be due to pregnancy.

Causal Factors

The most common cause of absence of withdrawal bleeding is inadequate development of the endometrium as a result of insufficient estrogen activity. Interaction of OCs with other drugs may be responsible for low estrogen activity (see Section 6).

Management

Women who fail to have withdrawal menses should be checked for pregnancy before they start the next cycle of active OCs.

Patients initiating OC use should be told of the possibility that menses may fail to occur even if they are not pregnant and that they should continue to take their OCs until a pregnancy test can be performed.

If a patient cannot return for an examination or pregnancy test, she should be instructed to stop taking OCs and use a barrier contraceptive method until a definite diagnosis can be made.

Pelvic ultrasound with measurement of endometrial thickness can help to make a diagnosis. Wall-to-wall endometrial thickness will be less than 5 mm if amenorrhea is due to lack of estrogen stimulation; endometrial thickness of less than 6 mm is incompatible with intrauterine pregnancy.

Changing OCs

Patients with absence of menses who are not pregnant may choose to:

22

- Continue taking the same OC and have no menses
- Switch to a different OC with the same amount of estrogen but with greater endometrial activity by lowering the progestin dose or changing to a different progestin
- Switch to a multiphasic OC
- Continue with the same OC and take additional estrogen tablets.

A switch to an OC with a higher estrogen dose (e.g., 50 mcg EE) is seldom necessary.

If patients choose to remain on the same OC despite the absence of menses, additional contraceptive measures are not necessary unless BTB occurs.

A switch to an OC with a higher estrogen content or an addition of estrogen tablets should be contemplated only after attempts to restore menses by switching to an OC with higher endometrial activity.

A higher estrogen content OC or adding estrogen tablets need be used only for one or two cycles before returning to a lower-dose OC. Continued use of higher estrogen OCs should be considered only after failure of all other measures to produce regular withdrawal bleeding.

DIETARY AND EXERCISE AMENORRHEA

Dietary and exercise amenorrhea are associated with low serum levels of FSH, LH, E2, T4, and increased levels of prolactin.

Careful histories and analyses of patients usually reveal total daily caloric intakes of less than 1,000 and carbohydrate intakes of less than 100 grams. Glucose tolerance tests

(GTTs) performed on patients with dietary amenorrhea will commonly return to fasting levels one hour after the glucose challenge.

Dietary amenorrhea is often resistant to ovarian stimulation with menopausal gonadotropins. Ovulation frequently resumes after food intake is increased to 1,800 calories per day with at least 200 grams of carbohydrates.

If amenorrhea is due to excessive exercise, FSH and thyroid levels will be low normal and prolactin levels may initially be slightly elevated. Menses may resume when caloric intake is increased and/or exercise is decreased.

POST-PILL AMENORRHEA/
AMENORRHEA AND GALACTORRHEA

Failure to resume menses within six weeks of discontinuing OC is referred to as post-pill amenorrhea (PPA). Amenorrhea after stopping OC with galactorrhea (the abnormal discharge of milk or fluid from the breast sometimes only detectable by squeezing the nipple) is referred to as PPAG.

Clinical Information

When high-estrogen content OCs were first introduced in the early 1960s, PPA and PPAG were frequent sequelae of OC use. Amenorrhea was usually self-limiting and could last for up to 12 months but usually lasted no more than three months. As estrogen doses were lowered, PPA and PPAG occurred less frequently and are now rarely seen (1, 2, 3).

PPAG after discontinuing OC use may be the result of (4):

- Hyperplasia of lactotrope cells/increased prolactin (15.7%)
- A prolactin or growth hormone-secreting pituitary adenoma (6.7%)
- Hypothalamic deficiency (51.2%).

Pituitary adenomas may be present in up to 24% of PPAG patients, whereas its incidence in patients with spontaneously occurring amenorrhea with galactorrhea is 55%. There is no evidence that OC users are more likely to develop pituitary adenomas than nonusers.

Other causes for failing to resume menstruating immediately after discontinuing OCs include:
- Pregnancy
- Hypothyroidism
- Polycystic ovaries (PCO)
- Ovarian failure/menopause
- Physiological factors, e.g., starvation, excessive exercise
- Obesity (weight gain greater than 30 lbs.)
- Psychological factors (e.g., anorexia)
- Use of psychotropic drugs (5)
- Non-prolactin or growth hormone-producing pituitary adenoma
- Any factors causing PPAG.

Women (except those with PCO) who had irregular menses before taking OCs are more likely to have amenorrhea after discontinuing OC use.

PCO patients may have one or two regular ovulatory cycles and may become pregnant immediately after discontinuing OCs before resuming their pre-OC patterns of menses every three to six months.

Amenorrhea that occurs during OC use is frequently due to inadequate hormone content or pregnancy.

Causal Factors for Amenorrhea and Galactorrhea

Estrogen present in OCs stimulates prolactin secretion by a direct action on pituitary lactotroph cells.

Prolactin prevents ovulation and menstruation by inhibiting gonadotropin-releasing hormone (GnRH) production by the hypothalamus and by blocking the ovarian response to luteinizing hormone (LH).

Use of psychotropic drugs may lead to increased prolactin production by blocking the production or action of dopamine, a natural prolactin inhibitor in the central nervous system. These drugs include reserpin, phenothiazines, and tricyclic antidepressants (see (6) for complete list).

Primary hypothyroidism results in high levels of TSH, which directly stimulates prolactin production by the lactotrope cells.

Management

When PPAG is diagnosed, evaluation should proceed at once, starting with serum prolactin.

Serum prolactin levels may be interpreted as follows:

- 35 µg/ml—Prolactin-secreting tumor not present
- 36 to 50 µg/ml—Probable lactotrophe hyperplasia but possible prolactin-secreting tumor; prolactin levels should be repeated in six months
- 50 to 200 µg/ml—Higher probability of prolactinemia:
  - A pituitary serial tomogram, CAT scan, or MRI is indicated; if these are negative, prolactin levels should be repeated every six to 12 months
  - Tomograms and CAT scans should be repeated only if prolactin levels rise (cataracts may result from repeated use)
- Greater than 200 µg/ml - Probable pituitary adenoma:
  - A pituitary scan is needed

If PPA is the only symptom, it is acceptable to wait for spontaneous return of menses after elimination of possible causes, e.g.:

- Pregnancy
- Pituitary disorders
- Thyroid disease
- Psychotropic drug use
- Menopause

Patients should use barrier methods if they desire contraception while waiting for spontaneous resumption of menses.

Women with pre-existing amenorrhea prior to OC use should be advised of the possibility that amenorrhea may return after they discontinue OC use and should be encouraged to use other contraceptive methods.

Treatment of Elevated Prolactin

Bromocriptine (Parlodel®, Sandoz) is the first medical treatment for patients with prolactin-secreting tumors and those with pituitary hyperplasia and amenorrhea who desire pregnancy. Side effects of bromocriptine are reduced if one-half a tablet is taken every eight hours instead of one tablet every 12 hours. Other drugs that can be taken orally daily, e.g., peroglide mesylate (Permax®), or twice weekly, e.g., cabergolise (Dostinex®), are now more commonly used.

Menses resumes in an average of five weeks after beginning therapy for hyperprolactinemia, but may be delayed for several months if prolactin levels are high. Patients who fail to ovulate with prolactin-suppressing drugs alone may respond when clomiphene citrate 50 to 100 mg daily for five days is added.

After menses is re-established, prolactin-suppressing drugs may only be needed for the first two weeks of each cycle, thereby avoiding medication after conception has occurred.

References for Section 22: Amenorrhea

1. Dickey RP: Treatment of post-pill amenorrhea. Int J Gynecol Obstet 1977;15:125–132.
2. Dickey RP, Berger GS: Persistent amenorrhea and galactorrhea. In: Clinical Use of Sex Steroids. Givens JR (ed.) Chicago: Yearbook Medical Publishing, 1980;329–388.
3. Josimovich JB et al.: Heterogeneous distribution of serum prolactin values in apparently healthy young women and the effects of oral contraceptive medication. Fertil Steril 1987;47:785.
4. Pituitary Adenoma Study Group. Pituitary adenomas and oral contraceptives: A multicenter case control study. Fertil Steril 1983;39(6):753–760.
5. Federal Drug Administration Drug Bulletin. April 1990;5.
6. Dickey RP, Stone SC: Drugs that affect the breast and lactation. Clin Obstet Gynecol 1975;18:2.

SECTION 23: UTERINE CHANGES AND OVARIAN CHANGES

UTERINE CHANGES

Leiomyomas (Fibroids)
Clinical Information

Uterine size and the size of pre-existing leiomyomas may increase or decrease, depending on the estrogen activity of a particular OC and the sensitivity of the individual woman (1). Uterine fibroids are reduced in size and number in current OC users but not in former users (2).

Cellular atypia may occur in leiomyomas of OC users (3). However, a definite relationship between OC hormones and atypical leiomyomas has not been demonstrated. Leiomyomas with multifocal hemorrhages (apoplectic leiomyomas) may be more common in OC users (4). Symptoms usually develop after two to four years of OC use. Pain may be sufficient to require laparotomy.

The incidence of newly discovered fibroids decreases with years of OC use but returns to control levels after OCs are discontinued (5).

Causal Factors

The myometrium is one of the most sensitive tissues to the stimulation of estrogen. Estrogen causes both a real growth of myometrial cells and edema.

Many progestins antagonize the effect of estrogen and cause a real decrease in leiomyoma size.

Endometrial Cancer

The risk of developing endometrial cancer is reduced 50% after one year of OC use, decreases further with increasing length of use, and continues to be reduced for at least 15 years after discontinuing OCs (6, 7, 8, 9, 10, 11). This protection extends to adenocarcinoma, adenoacanthoma, and adenosquamous lesions. Protection has been reported for all monophasic OCs, including those with less than 50 mcg EE.

164

Thus far, insufficient data have been collected on multiphasic OCs to determine if they also provide protection.

The risk of endometrial cancer in both users and nonusers is low. A meta-analysis estimated that the risk of nonusers developing endometrial cancer through age 74 was 2.4% compared with 1.4% for women who had used OCs for 12 years (12,13). One analysis estimated that use of OCs for eight years or longer would result in 1,900 fewer cases of endometrial cancer in the U.S. (14). However, another researcher estimated that, for 100,000 women who used OCs continuously from ages 16 to 35, there would be only 10 fewer deaths from endometrial cancer over their lifetimes (15).

23

OVARIAN CHANGES
(See Section 2 for discussion of polycystic ovaries)

Clinical Information

The incidence of benign ovarian cysts is reduced in OC users. However, there are several reports of the development of follicular and corpus luteum cysts, some very large, in patients using triphasic and low-dose monophasic OCs (2, 16, 17). In all cases in which patients switched to high-progesterone potency monophasic OCs, the cysts resolved.

In a randomized, controlled study, the risk of developing a functional ovarian cyst (larger than 3.0 mm) during OC use was twice as high for low-dose monophasic and triphasic OCs than for higher-dose monophasic OCs (18). A shorter pill-free interval may decrease the incidence of functional cysts in women taking low-dose or multiphasic OCs (19).

Ovarian Cancer

The incidence of ovarian cancer is reduced in OC users. This protective effect increases with years of use from 14% after one year to 50 to 60% after five years (12, 20, 21, 22). Protection is greatest in women younger than age 25. The risk reduction is the same in women who use low-estrogen <50 mcg EE/low progestin OCs as for those who used high estrogen ≥ 50 mcg EE/high progestin OCs (23). The risk reduction occurs with all monophasic OCs and extends to serous, endometrial, and clear cell tumors (12). It is uncertain if mucinous and other benign tumors are prevented (24). This reduced risk appears to persist for as long as 10 years after discontinuing OC use.

OCs reduce the risk of hereditary ovarian cancer to the same extent for women with either the BRCA1 or the BRCA2 mutations as for noncarriers. In carriers, the risk was reduced 60% in women taking OCs for six years or longer (25).

A 1995 meta-analysis estimated the risk of developing ovarian cancer in never-users ages 20 to 54 to be 369 per 100,000 women. For women using OCs for eight years, the estimated risk was decreased by 193 cases (26). Another analysis estimated that the number of cases of ovarian cancer per 100,000 U.S. women would be decreased by 215 cases over their lifetimes if they used OCs for five years (20).

Management

OCs are important in the management of many types of benign ovarian cysts. Benign ovarian cysts include:
- Hemorrhagic cysts
- Simple cysts
- Cysts resulting from use of ovulation induction drugs
- Endometriomas.

All ovarian cysts larger than 4 cm should be considered as potential neoplasm, and appropriate steps leading to laparoscopic or surgical exploration should be instituted.

Cysts smaller than 4 cm that have no malignant characteristics with ultrasound may be initially managed by a trial of OC suppression. The most effective OCs for this purpose are the high progestational activity OCs Ogestrel® and Ovral® (0.5 mg NG/50 mcg EE). Cysts should decrease in volume by at least 50% in 21 days (this may represent only a 20-percent decrease in diameter). Cysts that do decrease in volume should be considered malignant until proven otherwise. However, endometriomas may also fail to decrease by 50% in volume.

Hemorrhagic corpus luteum cysts may initially appear similar to endometriomas on ultrasound but will be suppressed by high-progestational activity OCs. They are often recurrent and can lead to repeated hospitalizations and possible ovarian adhesions. Recurrence of hemorrhagic corpus luteum cysts may be prevented by prophylactic use of combination OCs with intermediate progestational activity.

Simple (unilocular cysts) of the ovary usually result from preovulatory follicles that contain an atretic oocyte. These can grow to become 4 cm in size and persist into the next cycle. Simple cysts are often recurrent and are more common at the extremes of reproductive life, a time when malignant cysts are also more common. Spontaneous resolution may occur in 50% of simple cysts within 60 days (27). Simple cysts that do not resolve spontaneously may be treated initially with high-progestational activity OCs, or with intermediate to high progestational activity monophasic OCs (see Table 9). Cyclic use of intermediate to high progestational activity monophasic OC will prevent recurrence of cysts in most patients.

In one report, 73% of adnexal cysts were resolved during six weeks of OC treatment. Adnexal pathology was present at surgery in the remaining patients (19).

OCs may be used in the cycle prior to ovulation induction with hMG or follicle-stimulating hormone. OCs with intermediate progestational and estrogenic activities (1 mg norethindrone and 35 mcg EE) should be used because excessively high progestational and/or estrogenic activities will inhibit follicle development in the following cycle.

OC suppression of ovarian cysts can be started on the first day of menstruation in regularly cycling patients. OCs may be started at any time after ruling out pregnancy in non-cycling patients.

References for Section 23: Uterine Changes and Ovarian Changes

1. Friedman AJ, Thomas PP: Does low-dose combination oral contraceptive use affect uterine size or menstrual flow in premenopausal women with leiomyomas? Obstet Gynecol 1995;85:631- 635.

2. Chiaffarino Francesca et al.: Oral contraceptive use and benign gynecologic conditions. Contraception 1998;57:11–18.

3. Fechner RE: The surgical pathology of the reproductive system and breast during oral contraceptive therapy. Pathol Ann 1971;6: 299–319.

4. Myles JL, Hart WR: Apoplectic leiomyomas of the uterus: A clinicopathologic study of five distinctive hemorrhagic leiomyomas associated with oral contraceptive usage. Am J Surg Pathol 1985;9(11):798–805.

5. Chiaffarino Francesca et al.: Use of oral contraceptives and uterine fibroids: Results from a case-control study. Br J Obstet Gynaecol 1999;August (106):857–680.

6. CASH and NICH. Combination oral contraceptive use and the risk of endometrial cancer. JAMA 1987;257:796–800.

7. Jick SS, Walker AM, Jick H: Oral contraceptives and endometrial cancer. Obstet Gynecol 1993;82:931–935.

8. Kaufman DW et al.: Decreased risk of endometrial cancer among oral contraceptive users. N Engl J Med 1980;303:1045.

9. Silverberg SG, Makowski EL, Roche WD: Endometrial carcinoma in women under 40 years of age: Comparisons of cases in oral contraceptive users and nonusers. Cancer 1977;39:592–598.

10. Thomas DB: The WHO collaborative study of neoplasia and steroid contraceptives: The influence of combined oral contraceptives or risk of neoplasms in developing and developed countries. Contraception 1991;43:695–710.

11. Weiss NS, Sayvetz TA et al.: Incidence of endometrial cancer in relation to oral contraceptives. N Engl J Med 1980;302:551.

12. Schlesselman JJ: Net effect of oral contraceptive use on the risk of cancer in women in the United States. Obstet Gynecol 1995;85: 793–801.

13. Schlesselman JJ: Risk of endometrial cancer in relation to use of combined oral contraceptives: A practitioner's guide to meta-analysis. Hum Reprod 1997;12:1851–1863.

14. Petitti DB, Porterfield D: Worldwide variations in the lifetime probablity of reproductive cancer in women: Implications of best case and worst case assumptions about the effect of oral contraceptive use. Contraception 1992;45:93–104.

15. Vessey MP et al.: Neoplasia of the cervix and uterus and contraception: A possible adverse effect of the pill. Lancet 1983;2: 930–934.

16. Caillouette JC, Koehler AL: Phasic contraceptive pills and functional ovarian cysts. Am J Obstet Gynecol 1987;156:1538–1542.

17. Ylikorkala O: Ovarian cysts and hormonal contraception. Lancet 1977;1:1101–1102.

18. Grimes DA, Godwin AJ, Rubin A, Smith JA, Lacarra M: Ovulation and follicular development associated with three low-dose oral contraceptives: A randomized controlled trial. Obstet Gynecol 1994;83:29–34.

19. Spanos WJ: Preoperative hormonal therapy of cystic adnexal masses. Am J Obstet Gynecol 1973;116:551.

20. Coker AL, Harlap S, Fortney JA: Oral contraceptives and reproductive cancers: Weighing the risks and benefits. Fam Plann Perspect 1993;25:17–21.

21. Franceschi S, Parazzini F, Negri E, et al.: Pooled analysis of three European case control studies of epithelial ovarian cancer: III. Oral contraceptive use. Int J Cancer 1991;49:61–65.

22. Heintz APM, Hacker NF, Lagasse LD: Epidemiology and etiology of ovarian cancer: A review. Obstet Gynecol 1985;66:127–135.

23. Ness RB, Grisso JA, Klapper J, Schlesselman JJ, Solberzweig S, Vergona R, Morgan M, Wheeler JE and the SHARE Study Group. Risk of ovarian cancer in relation to estrogen and progestin dose and use characteristics of oral contraceptives. Am J Epidemiol 2000;152:233–41.

24. Westhoff C, Britton JA, Gammon MD, Wright T, Kelsey JL. Oral contraceptives and benign ovarian tumors. Am J Epidemiol 2000;152:242–6.

25. Morris JM, Van Wagenen G: Interception: The use of postovulatory estrogens to prevent implantation. Am J Obstet Gynecol 1973;115:101–106.

26. Royal College of General Practitioners Oral Contraceptive Study. Further analysis of mortality in oral contraceptive users. Lancet 1981;1:541.

27. Bailey CL, Ueland FR, Land GL, DePriest PD, Gallion HH, Kryscio RJ, van Nagell JR Jr.: The malignant potential of small cystic ovarian tumors in women over 50 years of age. Gynecol Oncol 1998;69:3–7.

SECTION 24: VAGINAL CHANGES AND CERVICAL CHANGES

VAGINAL CHANGES

Clinical Information

Vaginal infections that may be increased in OC users include (1, 2):

- Vaginitis
- Vulvitis
- Moniliasis (yeast, fungus)
- Trichomoniasis
- HIV-1.

Vaginitis, vulvitis, and moniliasis have been reported as increased in OC users in some studies. The incidence of trichomoniasis is unchanged or decreased by OC use.

Leukorrhea, or mucoid discharge identical to the egg white-like discharge that precedes ovulation, is sometimes noted with high-estrogenic activity OCs.

OC users had twice the incidence of moniliasis in a Royal College of General Practitioners study (3).

All form of hormonal contraception, OCs, Injections, and Implants, have been shown to reduce the incidence of Bacterial Vaginosis compared to condoms and sterilization, in non-pregnant women attending a birth control clinic (Ob.Gyn. News September 1,2003)

Pelvic inflammatory disease (PID) is significantly decreased in OC users (4). However, OCs do not offer any protection against sexually transmitted diseases, such as herpes genitalis.

HIV-1-infected cells were significantly increased in endocervical and vaginal swabs from patients who used Depo-Provera® (odds ratio [OR] = 2.9) and both low-dose (OR = 3.8) and high-dose (OR = 12.3) OCs (5). Vitamin A was also associated with increased vaginal HIV-1 shedding in the same study.

Management

Mucoid discharge, especially when cervical hypertrophy is also present, can be treated by switching patients to OCs with less estrogenic activities.

Persistent or recurrent vaginitis, moniliasis, or other local infections may necessitate a switch to an OC with lower progestational activity.

Herpes genitalis is not related to OC use. No specific treatment is known. Nonoxynol and related drugs used *in vitro* in vaginal spermicidal products are toxic to herpes genitalis.

The contraceptive effectiveness of OCs is reduced with use of metronidazole for treatment of trichomoniasis and other infections (6); therefore, additional contraceptive measures should be used during this treatment regimen.

If cervical hypertrophy or ectopy occurs, patients should be switched to OCs with lower estrogenic activities. If repeated cervicitis occurs, patients should be switched to OCs with lower progestational and androgenic activities.

CERVICAL CHANGES

Cervicitis
Clinical Information

Chlamydia trachomatis, endocervicitis, is more common in OC users. At the same time, the incidence of symptomatic PID is decreased (7, 8, 9).

Causal Factors

Use of OCs is associated with increased cervical ectopy (endocervical cells advancing onto the ectocervix) (10). Endocervical cells are the primary sites for attachment of Chlamydia. trachomatis and Neisseria gonorrhea.

Cervical hypertrophy and ectopy are due to the estrogen components of OCs and result from accelerated growth of endocervical cells on to the exterior of the cervix. Cervicitis is related to the progestin content.

Management

Use of newer low-dose combination and triphasic OCs may reduce the incidence of cervical ectopy.

Cervical Cancer

Clinical Information

There is evidence of a relationship between OC use and a small increase in cervical cancer (11, 12, 13, 14, 15, 16, 17, 18, 19, 20, 21).

A 2003 meta-analysis of 28 studies involving 12,531 women with cervical cancer investigated the relationship between invasive and *in situ* cervical cancer and duration and recency of OC use with particular attention to human papilloma virus (HPV) infection (21). The relative risk of cervical cancer increased with increasing duration of OC use. Compared to nonusers, the RR was < 5 yrs 1.1, 5–9 yrs 1.6, > 10 yrs. 2.2. Results were broadly similar for invasive and *in situ*, for squamous cell and adenocarcinoma, and in studies that adjusted for HPV status, number of sexual partners, smoking, and use of barrier contraceptives. HPV status did not appear to add to the risk.

A 1995 meta-analysis estimated the risk of developing cervical cancer for ages 20 to 54 to be 425 per 100,000 women years in nonusers. It estimated that an additional 125 cases might occur in women who used OCs for eight or more years (18). Another analysis estimated that use of OCs for eight years or longer would result in 30 additional cases of cervical cancer in the U.S. (16). Yet another analysis estimated that the number of cases of cervical cancer per 100,000 U.S. women would be increased by 67 cases during their lifetimes if they used OCs for five years (22). A further researcher estimated that, for 100,000 women who used OCs continuously from ages 16 to 35, there would be an additional 76 deaths from cervical cancer during their lifetimes (23).

There has been a greater than twofold increase in adenocarcinoma of the cervix between the early 1970s and mid-1980s in women younger than age 35. One case-control study found a relative risk of 2.1 for adenocarcinoma of the cervix in users of OCs compared to nonusers (24). The risk was highest (4.4-fold) with use for longer than 12 years. No additional risk was found for age at first use.

The increased risk of cervical cancer has to be balanced against a 50-percent decrease in endometrial and ovarian cancers.

Causal Factors

The small increase in incidence of cervical cancer may be associated with increased susceptibility to the papilloma virus (25). Cervical lesions associated with the human papilloma virus and underlying stromal cells contain significantly more progesterone and estrogen receptors than normal cervical cells or stromal cancer (26).

The primary risk factors for cervical cancer are early sexual activity and multiple partners.

Management

Annual pap smears should be performed in women who use or have used OCs for more than five years (27). Women suspected of having cancer should be evaluated without regard to OC use.

Women with proven cancer should discontinue OC use because of the increased risk of thromboembolism and the possibility of accelerated tumor growth. Other methods of birth control should be recommended for these women.

References for Section 24: Vaginal Changes and Cervical Changes

1. Peddie BA et al.: Relationship between contraceptive method and vaginal flora. Austral NZ J Ob Gyn 1984;24:217.
2. Walnut Creek Contraceptive Drug Study. Results of the Walnut Creek Contraceptive Drug Study. J Repro Med 1980;25(suppl):346.
3. Royal College of General Practitioners. Oral contraceptives and health: An interim report from the oral contraception study of the Royal College of General Practitioners. New York: Pitman, 1974.
4. Senanayake P, Kramer DG: Contraception and the etiology of PID: New perspectives. Am J Obstet Gynecol 1980;138:852–860.

5. Mostad SB, Overbaugh J, DeVange DM, Welch MJ, Chohan B, Mandaliya K, Nyange P, Martin HL, Ndinya-Achola J, Bwayo JJ, Kreiss JK: Hormonal contraception, vitamin A deficiency, and risk factors for shedding of HIV-1 infected cells from the cervix and vagina. Lancet 1997;350:922–927.

6. Jimenez J et al.: Long-term follow-up of children breastfed by mothers receiving depomedroxyprogesterone acetate. Contraception 1984;30(6):523–533.

7. Blum M, Gilerovitch M, Benaim J, Appelbaum T: The correlation between chlamydia antigen, antibody, vaginal colonization, and contraceptive method in young, unmarried women. Adv Contracept 1990;6:41–45.

8. McGregor JA, Hammill HA: Contraceptive and sexually transmitted disease: Interactions and opportunities. Am J Obstet Gynecol 1993;168:2033–2041.

9. Svensson L, Westrom L, Mardh PA: Contraceptives and acute salpingitis. JAMA 1984;251:2553–2555.

10. Goldacre MJ, Loudon N, Watt B, et al.: Epidemiology and clinical significance of cervical erosion in women attending a family planning clinic. Br Med J 1978;1:748–750.

11. Andolsek L et al.: Influence of oral contraceptives on the incidence of premalignant and malignant lesions of the cervix. Contraception 1983; 28(6):505–529.

12. Brinton LA: Oral contraceptives and cervical neoplasia. Contraception 1991;43:581–595.

13. Brinton LA et al.: Long-term use of oral contraceptives and risk of invasive cervical cancer. Int J Cancer 1986;38(3):339–344.

14. Herbst AL, Berek JS: Impact of contraception on gynecologic cancers. Am J Obstet Gynecol 1993;168:1980–1985.

15. Khoo SK: Cancer risks and the contraceptive pill: What is the evidence after nearly 25 years of use? Med J Auth 1986;144(4): 185–190.

16. Petitti DB, Porterfield D: Worldwide variations in the lifetime probablity of reproductive cancer in women: Implications of best case and worst case assumptions about the effect of oral contraceptive use. Contraception 1992;45:93–104.

17. Piper JM: Oral contraceptives and cervical cancer. Gynecol Oncol 1985;22(1):1–14.

18. Schlesselman JJ: Net effect of oral contraceptive use on the risk of cancer in women in the United States. Obstet Gynecol 1995;85: 793–801.

19. Thomas DB: The WHO collaborative study of neoplasia and steroid contraceptives: The influence of combined oral contracep-

tives or risk of neoplasms in developing and developed countries. Contraception 1991;43:695–710.

20. Valente PT, Hanjani P: Endocervical neoplasia in long-term users of oral contraceptives: Clinical and pathologic observations. Obstet Gynecol 1986;67:695–704.

21. Smith JS, Green J, de Gonzalez AB, Appleby P, Peto J, Plummer M, Franceschi S, Beral V. Cervical cancer and use of hormonal contraceptives: a systematic review. Lancet 2003;361:1159–67.

22. Coker AL, Harlap S, Fortney JA: Oral contraceptives and reproductive cancers: Weighing the risks and benefits. Fam Plann Perspect 1993;25:17–21.

23. Vessey MP: The Jephcott Lecture, 1989: An overview of the benefits and risks of combined oral contraceptives. In: Mann RD, ed. Oral Contraceptives and Breast Cancer. Park Ridge, New Jersey: Parthenon 1989;121:35.

24. Ursin G, Peters RK, Henderson BE, d'Ablaing G, Monroe KR, Pike MC: Oral contraceptive use and adenocarcinoma of cervix. Lancet 1994;344:1390- 1394.

25. Bamford PN, Forbes-Smith PA, Rose GL, et al.: An analysis of factors responsible for progression or regression of mild and moderate cervical dyskaryosis. Br J Fam Plann 1985;11:5–8.

26. Vessey MP et al.: Neoplasia of the cervix and uterus and contraception: A possible adverse effect of the pill. Lancet 1983;2: 930–934.

27. Burslem RW: Cervical cytological screening for users of oral contraceptives. Lancet 1983;2:968.

SECTION 25: BREAST DISORDERS

BREAST SYMPTOMS

Clinical Information
Swelling and breast tenderness are common premenstrual symptoms and occur frequently in women using high estrogen- and high progestin-dose OCs. The incidence of breast symptoms seems to be decreased in women using low-dose formulations.

Causal Factors
Breast symptoms may be due to:
- Edema
- Growth of breast tissue
- Infection
- Vascular congestion
- Drugs that increase prolactin levels (1).

Management
When breast tenderness and swelling are unilateral and there are no palpable masses, switching patients to OCs with lower estrogen potencies or lower progestin contents is indicated. Patients should also be instructed to reduce their caffeine and sodium intakes. A diuretic may also provide temporary relief of symptoms.

If symptoms persist, further evaluation is required (2).

FIBROCYSTIC BREAST DISEASE

Clinical Information
Fibrocystic breast disease includes the following entities:
- Breast nodules
- Fibrocystic disease
- Fibroadenomas
- Fibroadenosis.

Management

When breast tenderness and swelling are unilateral and there are no palpable masses, switching patients to OCs with lower estrogen potencies or lower progestin contents is indicated. Patients should also be instructed to reduce their caffeine and sodium intakes. A diuretic may also provide temporary relief of symptoms.

If symptoms persist, further evaluation is required (2).

The incidence of benign nodules of the breast requiring breast biopsies (fibroadenosis and fibrocystic disease) was reduced 30% after one to two years of OC use and 50 to 65% after two years of use in two studies (3, 4). Other studies have not found OCs to be protective against the development of fibrocystic breast disease that requires breast biopsy (5, 6, 7, 8).

Women with fibrocystic breast disease may be at increased risk of developing breast cancer (9).

Causal Factors

Estrogen stimulates breast tissue growth directly by acting on the breast tissue (10), and indirectly by stimulation of prolactin production (2). Progestins antagonize these effects of the estrogen component. This antagonism is greatest in OCs with high progestational and/or androgenic activities.

Management

Women should be carefully monitored if they elect to use OCs and have strong family histories of:

- Breast nodules
- Fibrocystic disease
- Breast cancer.

Women who experience bilateral breast pain or masses without edema, while taking OCs, should be examined for malignancy by palpation and mammography. If no abnormalities are found, these women may be switched to OCs with lesser amounts of both estrogen and progestin.

If pain is due to edema, women should be switched to OCs with progestins that have less androgenic activities or lower estrogen doses.

If pain continues or if masses fail to decrease in size within one month, OCs should be discontinued.

BREAST CANCER

Clinical Information

A 1996 meta-analysis that included 53,297 women with breast cancer and 100,239 controls from 54 studies conducted in 25 countries concluded (11) that:

- There is a small increase in the relative risk (RR) of having breast cancer diagnosed while combined OCs are taken and for up to 10 years following discontinuance
- There is no increased excess risk of diagnosis 10 years or more after OCs are discontinued
- Cancers diagnosed in women who used combined OCs were less advanced clinically than cancers diagnosed in women who had not used OCs
- Breast cancers diagnosed in ever-users were less clinically advanced than those diagnosed in never-users for up to 20 years after discontinuing OCs.

In the same study, there was no significant variation in RR associated with specific types of estrogen or progestin. When grouped according to hormone dose, there was a decreased risk of diagnosed breast cancer with increasing estrogen dose among women who had discontinued use 10 years before. The authors concluded that these results were incompatible with a genotoxic effect, but were perhaps compatible with the concept that OCs may promote the growth of cancers already initiated. The authors also suggested that the decreased risk, seen in certain groups 10 years after OCs were discontinued, may be analogous to the protective effect of childbearing on breast cancer.

Previous Studies

Previous studies have shown either a slight increase in risk or a possible protective effect against breast cancer for

OC users, after adjusting for other risk factors risk. These studies reported either a slight increase in risk or a possible protective effect against breast cancer for OC users, after adjusting for other risk factors (48 references of studies on breast cancer and OC use were cited in the 9th edition). One review of 22 epidemiological studies found no increased risk in OC users. Another found no adverse effect on the progression of breast cancer among women taking OCs at the time of diagnosis.

Other Risk Factors

No positive relationship between breast cancer and caffeine use has been found, although a relationship to benign breast disease is known. Among subgroups of women who used OCs for more than four years and who developed breast cancer before age 36, the risk was increased for alcohol users vs nonusers (12). Another study, not as well controlled for additional risk factors, found the opposite effect, i.e., a decreased risk of breast cancer with alcohol use (13). A family history of breast cancer was also associated with increased risk (3.5 vs 1.43), while the risk was decreased with increasing body weight after adjustments for age at menarche, nulliparity, age at first term pregnancy, and/or breastfeeding (14).

Incidence

A 1995 meta-analysis estimated the risk of developing breast cancer from ages 20 to 54 in nonusers to be 2,782 per 100,000 women per years (WYS). For women using OCs for eight years, the estimated number of additional cases of breast cancer was 151 per 100,000 WYS (15). Another analysis estimated that the number of cases of breast cancer per 100,000 U.S. women would be increased by 134 cases over their lifetimes if they used OCs for five years (16). These potential increases must be balanced against a 50-percent decrease in endometrial and cervical cancers.

Causal Factors

The cause of breast cancer is unknown.

Women are known to be at increased risk of developing breast cancer if they:

- Have family histories of breast cancer in first-order relatives
- Have histories of biopsies for benign breast disease
- Are nulliparous or had first term pregnancies at ages 25 or older
- Achieved menarche before age 12
- Were not breastfed.

Women using combination OCs exhibited an increased frequency of sister-chromatid exchange in one study (17).

Pre-existing neoplasms may increase in size and become more easily noticed in some women after they start OCs. Conversely, breasts may become smaller in women taking low estrogen OCs, while nonhormone-sensitive neoplasms remain unchanged in size.

Management

Women with unilateral breast pain or discrete breast masses should discontinue OCs and use different contraceptive methods until a diagnosis of possible breast neoplasm is either confirmed or refuted. A breast mass that appears for the first time while OCs are being taken should be considered malignant until proven otherwise.

All women should have first mammograms upon reaching age 40 and screenings at one- to two-year intervals thereafter. Clinical breast examinations should be performed at least annually. Patients with symptoms of pain and change in breast size should be examined immediately.

Mammography is relatively insensitive for younger women. Only 45% of histologically confirmed breast cancers in women younger than age 36 with discrete masses were diagnosed by mammography compared to 78% diagnosed by fine needle aspiration (18).

In the same study, 16% of women with cancer had negative results on clinical examination, mammography, and fine needle aspiration. When all other investigations yield negative results, excision biopsy is mandatory in women with discrete breast masses.

Women at medium and high risks who are of low body weight and have strong family histories of breast cancer should be carefully monitored by breast examinations and mammograms, regardless of OC use.

Women younger than 36 who use OCs for more than four years, are of low body weight, and consume alcohol may be at additional risks for breast cancer.

It is still unclear whether OCs may be used safely by women who already have breast cancer despite two frequently cited studies that found no adverse effect on survival (19, 20).

Women diagnosed as having breast cancer while taking OCs may take some comfort in that their tumors are less likely to have spread and that earlier diagnosis may result in higher cure rates than occur for nonusers. Women who have not born children before age 30 may be encouraged by the speculation that OC use before age 30 may provide the same protective effect as having had a child (11).

References for Section 25: Breast Disorders

1. Dickey RP, Stone SC: Drugs that affect the breast and lactation. Clin Obstet Gynecol 1975;18:2.
2. Fechner RE: The surgical pathology of the reproductive system and breast during oral contraceptive therapy. Pathol Ann 1971;6:299–319.
3. Spanos WJ: Preoperative hormonal therapy of cystic adnexal masses. Am J Obstet Gynecol 1973;116:551.
4. Ory HW et al.: Oral contraceptives and reduced risk of benign breast diseases. N Engl J Med 1976;294:419–422.
5. Berkowitz GS et al.: Oral contraceptive use and fibrocystic disease among pre- and postmenopausal women. Am J Epidemiol 1984;120(1):87–96.
6. Franceschi S et al.: Oral contraceptives and benign breast disease: A case control study. Am J Obstet Gynecol 1984;149(6):602–606.
7. Hislop TG, Threlfall WJ: Oral contraceptives and benign breast disease. Am J Epidemiol 1984;120(2):273–280.

8. LiVolsi VA et al.: Fibrocystic disease in oral contraceptive users. N Engl J Med 1977;299:381.

9. Stadel BV, Schlesselman JJ: Oral contraceptive use and the risk of breast cancer in women with a prior history of benign breast disease. Am J Epidemiol 1986;123(3):373–382.

10. Hofseth LJ, Raafat AM, Osuch JR, Pathak DR, Slomski CA, Haslam SZ. Hormone replacement therapy with estrogen or estrogen plus medroxyprogesterone acetate is associated with increased epithelial proliferation in the normal postmenopausal breast. J Clin Endocrinol Metab 1999;84:4559–65.

11. Collaborative Group on Hormonal Factors in Breast Cancer. Breast cancer and hormonal contraceptives: Collaborative reanalysis of individual data on 53,297 women with breast cancer and 100,239 women without breast cancer from 54 epidemiological studies. Lancet 1996;347:1713–1727.

12. Longnecker MP et al.: A meta-analysis of alcohol consumption in relation to risk of breast cancer. JAMA 1988;260:652–656.

13. Graham S: Alcohol and breast cancer. N Engl J Med 1987;316: 1211–1313.

14. Kalache A, Vessey MP: Risks factors for breast cancer. In: Breast Cancer: Clinics of Oncology. Baum M (ed.) Philadelphia: WB Saunders, 1982.

15. Schlesselman JJ: Net effect of oral contraceptive use on the risk of cancer in women in the United States. Obstet Gynecol 1995;85:793–801.

16. Coker AL, Harlap S, Fortney JA: Oral contraceptives and reproductive cancers: Weighing the risks and benefits. Fam Plann Perspect 1993;25:17–21.

17. Murthy PBK, Prema K: Further studies on sister-chromatid exchange frequency in users of hormonal contraceptives. Mutat Res 1983;119(3):351–354.

18. Yelland A, Graham MD, Trott PA, Ford HT, Coombes RC, Gazet JC, Polson NG: Diagnosing breast carcinoma in young women. Br Med J 1991;302:618–620.

19. Henderson BE, Ross RK, Pike MC: Hormonal chemoprevention of cancer in women. Science 1993;259:633–638.

20. Rosner D, Lane WW: Oral contraceptive use has no adverse effect on the prognosis of breast cancer. Cancer 1986;57(3):591–596.

NOTES

SECTION 26:
CARDIOVASCULAR SYSTEM

GENERAL INFORMATION

Clinical Information

Cardiovascular disease (CVD) may be due to:
- Clotting within vessels e.g.:
  - Deep vein thrombosis
  - Pulmonary embolism
- Atherosclerotic changes within vessel walls e.g.:
  - Hypertension
  - Ischemic heart disease
- A combination of clotting and atherosclerotic effects, resulting in:
  - Myocardial infarction (MI)
  - Cerebrovascular accidents (CVA).

Virtually all the excess mortality in OC users is due to CVD (1). Early studies involving OCs with 50 to 150 mcg mestranol found a high incidence of CVD in OC users compared to nonusers (20 references were cited in the 9th edition). However, more recent studies involving OCs with 20 to 35 mcg EE and progestins with lower doses and less androgenic activities show a smaller increase and, in some cases, no increase in current or former OC users—except for women with specific risk factors (e.g., smoking, hypertension, obesity, and hereditary thrombophilia) (2, 3). The relationship of OCs to CVD has been the subject of several recent reviews (4, 5, 6, 7).

Causal Factors

CVD morbidity and deaths from both venous and nonvenous causes are related to the estrogen content (4, 8). OCs containing 30 mcg estrogen have lower morbidity rates than those with 50 mcg estrogen, which have lower rates than OCs containing more than 50 mcg estrogen (9).

Cardiovascular deaths are also related to the progestin dose and activity (4). Death and morbidity rates from all forms of CVD and stroke increase as the progestin dose increases from 1 to 2.5 mg norethindrone acetate and from 0.3 to 0.5 mg NG.

Estrogens, especially doses above 50 mcg EE, induce changes in coagulation and fibrolytic enzyme systems. Nearly all studies note an increase in plasma fibrinogen concentration and Factors II (prothrombin), VII, VIII, and X (10). These effects are questionable in OCs containing 20 mcg EE. Little difference in effects is shown between monophasic and multiphasic preparations with equal total estrogen contents.

One unconfirmed study found that Factor VII and X levels are significantly elevated in patients using 0.15 mg desogestrel and 0.075 mg gestodene with 30 mcg EE but not in patients using 0.15 mgdesogestrel with 20 mcg EE (11).

Progestins with higher androgenic activities increase the rate of atherosclerotic vascular changes by causing a decrease in plasma levels of high-density lipoprotein- (HDL) cholesterol, the cholesterol type that protects against arteriosclerotic vascular disease. Estrogen increases HDL-cholesterol levels. The effect of an OC on HDL-cholesterol depends on the type of progestin and the ratio of progestin-to-estrogen (see Table 7).

Other progestin-related changes with the potential to induce atherosclerotic vessel changes include increased levels (12) of:

- Total cholesterol
- Triglycerides
- Low-density lipoprotein (LDL)-cholesterol
- Very low-density lipoprotein (VLDL)-cholesterol.

Lower rates of venous thromboembolism (VTE), but higher rates of acute myocardial infarction for second-generation progestins (LNG and NG) compared to third-generation progestins (desogrestrel and gestodene), may be due to the antiestrogenic effect of the more androgenic, second-generation progestins rather than to any VTE-promoting effect of third-generation progestins (see Table 4).

26.

185

Women of Northern European descent have the highest incidence of venous thromboembolism (VTE), due in part to an increased incidence of Leiden factor V mutation. Women of African and Middle Eastern descent have a higher incidence of hypertension. Women of Asian descent have a lower incidence progestational and androgenic side effects (13).

Persistence of Risk of Vascular Disease CVD
Ethnic Differences

A 1981 prospective British study involving mostly OCs with greater than 50 mcg estrogen estimated that former users have a 2.6 times greater risk for all CVD than nonusers and that this risk remains elevated for at least six years after OCs are discontinued (see Table 16) (14).

Recent studies involving lower doses of EE and progestin show no increased risk of CVD after discontinuing OCs (5, 6, 15).

Reducing the Risk of CVD

The risk of CVD is reduced if OCs containing 35 mcg or less of estrogen and 0.5 mg or less of norethindrone or an equivalent amount of other progestins are used (see Tables 6 and 9).

OCs should not be prescribed for women who have the following conditions:
- Age 35 and older who smoke cigarettes
- Obesity of more than 10% over ideal weight
- Hypertension
- Current or past histories of thrombophlebitis
- Current hospitalization
- Immobilization of an extremity
- Family histories of CVA, MI, or pulmonary embolism before age 50
- Family histories of thrombophlebitis during pregnancy or OC use.

Several large family planning programs require that women older than age 35 and those with family histories of heart attack before age 50 have annual blood cholesterol,

186

triglyceride, and glucose determinations. Increased risk is present with levels of:

- Cholesterol—267 mg per 100 ml or higher
- Triglyceride—207 mg per 100 ml or higher
- Fasting glucose—105 mg per 100 ml or higher.

ACUTE MYOCARDIAL INFARCTION

Clinical Information

In some recent studies involving women who used sub-50 mcg OCs that contain the third-generation progestins desogestrel and gestodene, the incidence and mortality from acute myocardial infarction (AMI) were no different than for nonusers (see Table 17) (5, 16). For OCs containing the second-generation progestins levonorgestrel and sometimes norethindrone, the incidence and mortality of AMI were higher than for nonusers or third-generation OC users (5, 6, 15, 16, 17, 18, 19, 20, 21). When estrogen levels were less than 50 mcg, there was no increased risk of AMI after stopping OCs for either second- or third-generation progestin use.

Three recent studies comparing generations of OC progestins found basically identical results (22, 23, 24). Compared to non-OC users, the risk of MI for first generation progestins (norethindrone) current OC users was increased 2.2 (22) to 2.8 (23) times, the risk of MI for current second generation OC users was increased 2.2 (22), 2.4 (23), and 2.9 (24) times, while the risk of MI for third generation progestin OC users was either not increased 0.9 (24) or increased 1.3 (22, 23) times. The absolute risk of MI due to OC use is very low for young women, <1 case per 100,000, but rises to 30 cases per 100,000 among women 40–44 (7).

The apparent lower incidence of AMI with OCs containing third-generation progestins compared to OCs containing older progestins must be balanced against an apparent increase in deep vein thrombosis for third-generation progestins (19, 20, 25, 26). At a time when most OCs contained greater than 50 mcg estrogen, the mortality rate from AMI was much higher in current users and former users than in never users (see Table 16) (25 references were cited in the

9th edition). In contrast, an updated analysis of the long-running Oxford Family Planning Association study that comprised 17,000 women found OCs were associated with an increased risk of AMI only in heavy smokers. For this group, the relative risk was 4.9 for current OC users and 4.0 for former users (27).

Causal Factors

The incidence and mortality of AMI in OC users are related to the estrogen dose and type of progestin (i.e., estrogen/progestin balance) (9). Eighty percent of cases of AMI are related to smoking. The incidence of AMI could be decreased by 75% if all women of reproductive age stopped smoking (28).

The effect of smoking on MI is greatest for first-generation progestins and lowest for third-generation progestins when used in combination OCs (29):

- First-generation progestin OCs odds-ratio (OR) = 19.5
- Second-generation progestin OCs-OR = 9.5
- Third-generation progestin OCs-OR = 3.8.

In the same study, there was no increased risk to OC users who were former smokers.

There is a demonstrated relationship between the number of cigarettes smoked per day and the risk of fatal or nonfatal MI (30).

Cigarettes Per Day	Times MI Risk Is Increased
Less than 15	1.2 times
15 to 24	4.1 times
More than 24	11.3 times

Decreased fibrinolytic activity in vessel walls has been demonstrated both in women who used OCs for more than five years and in women who were smoking more than 10 cigarettes per day, suggesting the possibility of a synergistic effect (31).

The relative risk (RR) of AMI is related to numerous factors besides OC use (32). The RR according to underlying risk factors is estimated as (29):

- Cigarette smoking—9.7 times
- Hypertension—3.3 times
- High cholesterol (Type II hyperlipidemia)—4.2 times
- Obesity (BMI):
  - BMI less than 20—1.0 times
  - BMI 20 to 24—1.7 times
  - BMI 25 to 29—3.7 times*
  - BMI greater than 29—4.8 times
- Diabetes—2.5 times
- History of pre-eclamptic toxemia
- Family history of MI—3.7 times
- Parity—2.8 times.

*BMI of 25 occurs with a weight of 145 for a height of 5'4"

The greater the number of underlying risk factors, the higher the risk of AMI among OC users as well as nonusers (33):

- One factor increased the risk four times
- Two factors increased the risk 10 times
- Three factors increased the risk 78 times.

In a transnational study, OR for MI was 1.07 when blood pressure was checked before prescribing OCs, compared to 2.76 when blood pressure was not checked before OCs were prescribed (29).

Management

The risk of MI can be reduced by use of sub-50 mcg EE OCs, especially if they contain third-generation progestins, and by not prescribing OCs for women with additional risk factors, particularly smoking, hypertension, diabetes, family history of MI, and obesity.

Clinicians who prescribe OCs must be aware of the possibility of MI in all women, not just OC users. Mortality and morbidity can be substantially reduced if treatment with thrombolytic agents is initiated within three hours of an MI (34).

189

CEREBROVASCULAR ACCIDENTS

Clinical Information

Cerebrovascular accidents (CVAs) include cerebral thrombosis (ischemic stroke) and cerebral hemorrhage (hemorrhagic stroke). The incidence of either type of CVA for OC users is currently very low (see Table 17) (5, 35, 36, 37, 38,39, 40, 41). The incidence of hemorrhagic stroke for ages 20 to 24 was no different than for nonusers (5). For ages 40 to 44, the incidence and mortality of hemorrhagic stroke were doubled for OC users compared to nonusers. For women using sub-50 mcg OCs, the incidence of ischemic stroke was increased 2.5-fold for OC users ages 20 to 24, from 2.0- to 5.0-fold for those ages 40 to 44, and was the same for second- and third-generation progestins. There was no increased risk of either type of CVA after stopping OCs when estrogen levels were less than 50 mcg (42).

In early studies involving 50 to 150 mcg estrogen OCs and higher progestin doses, the incidence and mortality from CVA of all types was increased for current and former OC users compared to nonusers (see Table 16) (24 references were cited in the 9th edition).

Other factors significantly increase the risk of stroke: A 1995 Danish study of women ages 15 to 44 who had ischemic strokes found the odds ratio (OR), adjusted by multivariate analysis, to be 5.4 for diabetes, 3.1 for hypertension, 2.8 for migraine, and 5.3 for previous noncerebral vascular thrombosis (43). The increased risk for stroke in women with these factors was the same in OC users and nonusers.

In a study of all women in Denmark (ages 15 to 44) who experienced CVAs during 1985 to 1989 (44), the risk of ischemic stroke was increased:

- 2.9% for 50 mcg estrogen OCs
- 1.8% for 30 to 40 mcg estrogen OCs
- 0.9% for progestin-only pills.

Hypertension is a major risk factor for ischemic stroke. Compared to nonusers of OCs who do not have hypertension, OC users with hypertension had 10-fold increased risk of ischemic stroke (45). These ratios did not change with age or years of use. Cigarette smoking increased the risk of CVA by 50% independently of OCs in this study (11).

In a 1996 case-control study, the crude incidence of ischemic stroke was increased for women who smoked, had hypertension or diabetes, were obese, or were of African-American descent; and the incidence of hemorrhagic stroke was increased for women with all these factors except obesity in the same study (42).

A 1998 update of the Oxford Family Planning Association study of 17,000 women found the relative risk of ischemic stroke in smokers who used OCs was 2.9 compared with smokers who do not use OCs (27). The risk did not persist in former OC users.

Smoking increases the risk of subarachnoid hemorrhage (46).

Data from the 1991 RCGP study found the adjusted OR for thrombotic stroke was 0.6 in women who used sub-50 mcg OCs and did not smoke (47).

CVAs are often preceded by persistent headache for weeks or months and/or by transient hemiparesis. CVAs are rarely precipitated by mild hypertension but may be caused by extreme hypertension.

See General Information, Causal Factors, above.

Management

Women who develop persistent headaches and/or transient hemiparesis while taking OCs should discontinue use immediately. Women with migraine headaches that worsen while taking OCs should discontinue OC use. Women with family histories of CVAs or stroke in close relatives or with personal histories of transient hemiparesis may be at increased risk of experiencing the same conditions if they take OCs.

Clinicians who prescribe OCs should be aware of the possibility of stroke in all patients, not just OC users, and should be prepared to respond promptly to patients who report symptoms or have evidence of stroke. Mortality and morbidity can be substantially reduced if treatment with thrombolytic agents is initiated within three hours (48).

VENOUS THROMBOEMBOLISM (VTE) AND THROMBOPHLEBITIS

Clinical Information

Venous thromboembolism (VTE) includes deep vein thrombophlebitis and pulmonary embolism. An increased risk of VTE in OC users is well established, but its importance in terms of OC-related mortality is small compared to AMI. Only 1 to 3% of VTE cases result in death.

In recent studies involving women using sub-50 mcg OCs, the incidence in mortality from VTE is much lower (see Table 17) (5, 17, 26, 49, 50, 51, 52, 53, 54, 55, 56). The mortality from VTE per 100,000 women years for OCs containing second-generation progestins (levonorgestrel, norgestrel) was 0.3 for ages 15 to 24 compared with 0.1 for nonusers and 0.6 for ages 35 to 44 compared with 0.2 for nonusers. For OCs containing third-generation progestins (desogestrel and gestodene), the mortality per 100,000 women years was 0.2 to 0.7 for ages 15 to 24 and 0.5 to 2.8 for ages 35 to 44.

The higher incidence of VTE with OCs containing third-generation progestins compared with OCs containing third-generation progestins and to OCs containing older progestins must be balanced against a lower rate of acute myocardial infarction (AMI) with third-generation progestins (19, 20, 25, 26).

In early studies involving 50 to 150 mcg estrogen OCs and higher progestin doses, the mortality rate per 100,000 women years from VTE was 2.7 for current OC users and 2.2 for former users (see Table 16) (37 references were cited in the 9th edition).

But in a 1997 study in which cases and controls were exactly matched for age, the OR for VTE in third- vs second-generation progestins was 0.8 (57). In a 1999 study of first-time OC users, the OR for VTE in third- vs second-generation progestins was 3.9 (58).

The main risk factors for VTE are age, obesity, family history, and Leiden factor V mutation (59, 60, 61, 62). Obesity increases the risk of VTE two to four times. Trauma, immobilization, surgery (63), and cancer increase the risk of VTE. The incidence of VTE during pregnancy and the puerperium is 60 to 80 per 100,000 women years.

The risk of VTE is higher in first-time OC users (64). Virtually all VTE occurs before the second year of use.

There is no increased risk of VTE in users of postcoital contraceptive pills (65).

Superficial thrombophlebitis of the leg is a relatively benign condition that is rarely fatal.

In a study in which cases and controls were exactly matched for age, the OR for VTE in third- vs second-generation progestins was 0.8 (66).

Causal Factors

The increased incidence of VTE is believed to be due to an increased rate of clot formation induced by estrogen. In addition, progestins may cause dilation of veins, which results in a slowing of the rate of blood flow.

Leiden factor V mutation is associated with an increased incidence of VTE, and is present in 5% of the general population, and up to 40% of patients with histories of VTE (62, 67). Other thrombophilias of protein C and S deficiency occur in the general population at 0.5%, and rises to 4% in patients with histories of VTE (68). Thrombophilias, especially Leiden factor V mutation, caused an eightfold increase in VTE. This rises to 30-fold in women who use OCs (62).

There are no differences between newer and older OCs with regard to their effects on blood clotting (69).

Management

Signs of superficial and deep vein thrombosis include:
- Pain to the touch, localized to an extremity
- Swelling
- Warmth

193

- Altered blood flow (detected by ultrasonography or dye injection).

An increased risk of VTE and thrombosis is well established in women using OCs.

OCs should be discontinued and other birth control methods used if VTE is suspected. A diagnosis should be established by clinical and radiological methods.

Deep vein thrombosis must be treated by anticoagulant therapy.

PULMONARY EMBOLISM

Clinical Information

In the 1960s, the excess mortality rate due to pulmonary embolism or stroke was 2.8 deaths annually per 100,000 OC users (see Table 16) (8, 70, 71, 72, 73, 74, 75). About 1–3% of recognized cases of pulmonary embolism result in death (7). Pulmonary embolism is now rare due to use of sub-50 mcg estrogen OCs (5, 76).

Pulmonary embolism is characterized by:
- Shortness of breath
- Chest pain
- Hemoptysis (coughing of blood).

Other, conditions may mimic the symptoms of pulmonary embolism, including:
- Pleurisy
- Spontaneous rupture of the lung
- Trauma to rib or cartilage
- Pneumonia.

Causal Factors

See Cardiovascular Disease, General Information, above.

Management

When pulmonary embolism is suspected because of any of the symptoms listed above, immediate steps to establish a

194

diagnosis must be taken, including chest x-rays and radiographic lung scans, if available.

Once the diagnosis is established, immediate anticoagulant therapy is necessary. Ligation of the vena cava may be required if repeated embolism occurs.

Patients with deep vein thrombosis should have baseline lung x-rays and be observed closely to detect symptoms of pulmonary embolism.

OCs should not be restarted in patients who have experienced deep vein thrombosis.

Superficial thrombophlebitis may be treated by:
- Bed rest
- Heat
- Elevation of the extremity
- Anti-inflammatory agents (optional).

The low incidence of Leiden factor V mutation and other thrombophilias in the general population make screening of all patients impractical (77). Screening may be indicated in women with personal or family histories of thrombosis.

Most patients survive if treatment is started early.

OTHER THROMBOSES

Pre- and Postoperative Thromboembolism

Combination OCs should be discontinued four weeks before and two weeks after elective surgery and during prolonged immobilization (78, 79). Other contraceptive methods should be used during these times.

Mesenteric Artery or Vein Thrombosis

Mesenteric artery thrombosis is only half as common as mesenteric vein thrombosis, but is twice as likely to cause death. In a review of 21 OC-related cases, the mortality was 50%. Abdominal pain was present in all patients for two or more weeks due to small bowel ischemia (80, 81, 82).

In addition to persistent abdominal pain, other symptoms may include:

195

- Fever
- Elevated white blood cell count
- Vomiting
- Diarrhea
- Bloody stools or hematemesis (depending on the location in the bowel).

An upper gastrointestinal series, with follow-through, will show a narrowing of a small bowel segment.

Splenic Artery Thrombosis
Only one case of splenic artery thrombosis in an OC user has been reported. The patient presented with upper left-quadrant pain of two weeks duration and leukocytosis of 14,000 (83). An uneventful recovery followed the patient's splenectomy.

Inferior Vena Cava Thrombosis
One case of thrombosis of the entire inferior vena cava and renal, pelvic, and femoral veins has been reported. The 24-year-old patient presented with a backache of 10 days duration and swelling of the lower extremities (80).

The diagnosis was made by computed tomography. The patient was successfully treated with heparin.

Hepatic Vein Thrombosis
At least 47 cases of hepatic vein thrombosis (Budd-Chiari syndrome) have been reported in OC users (84, 85). Survival was 50% in both surgically and medically treated patients with early diagnosis and treatment. The relative risk for OC users has been calculated as 2.4 compared to nonusers (86).

Symptoms are pain and abdominal swelling. Elevated alkaline phosphatase may be the only abnormal lab value.

Other reported hepatic vascular complications in OC users include (87):
- Portal vein thrombosis
- Periportal sinusoidal dilatation

196

- Hepatic arteriole intimal hyperplasia
- Focal hemorrhagic necrosis (88).

HYPERTENSION

Clinical Information

OC-related hypertension, when it occurs, is usually mild to moderate (10 to 20 mm Hg diastolic and 20 to 40 mm Hg systolic), and the hypertension is usually reversible within one to three months after OCs are discontinued. A few cases progressing to malignant hypertension have been reported.

Women who used OCs were six times more likely to develop hypertension than nonusers in early studies (18 references were cited in the 9th edition).

The probability of developing hypertension increases with age and duration of OC use (89). Hypertension is not limited to the first months of use and, in fact, may appear at any time during OC use. Hypertension will appear in 5% of those who take OCs for five years (90).

A recent study found OC use was an independent risk factor for uncontrolled blood pressure among hypertensive women using OC for more than 8 years in a logistic regression model after controlling for age, weight, and antihypertensive medication (91).

Diastolic pressure levels increased with duration of use (0.5 mm Hg per year) in one study (92).

Women with family histories of hypertension or toxemia in pregnancy are more likely to develop hypertension while using OCs. In such cases, the OC is believed to unmask an underlying prehypertensive condition.

No deaths from malignant hypertension among current users were reported in the most recent RCGP study (6).

Causal Factors

Hypertension in OC users appears to be associated with the progestin component and increases with increasing concentrations of progestins (73, 93). Elevated blood pressure has not been found in women taking estrogen for menopausal hormone replacement.

See also General Information, above.

Management

Mild increases in blood pressure may be treated initially by switching patients to OCs with lower progestin activities. Patients should allow three months for return to normal blood pressures. If hypertension continues, OCs should be stopped and alternative contraceptive methods considered.

Antihypertensive medications should not be used along with OCs because of the differing mechanisms of actions of the two drug types. Stopping either the medication or the OC might result in an unpredictable change in blood pressure.

References for Section 26: Cardiovascular System

1. Tietze C: New estimates of mortality associated with fertility control. Fam Plann Perspect 1977; 9(2):74–76.

2. Kay CR: Oral contraceptives and cancer. Lancet 1983;2: 1018–1021.

3. Pardthaisong T, Gray RH: The return of fertility following discontinuance of oral contraceptives in Thailand. Fertil Steril 1981;35: 532.

4. Carr BR, Ory H: Estrogen and progestin components of oral contraceptives: Relationship to vascular disease. Contraception 1997; 55:267–272.

5. Consensus Conference on Combination Oral Contraceptives and Cardiovascular Disease. Fertil Steril 1999;June(71)6(Suppl 3):1S-6S.

6. Rosenberg L, Palmer JR, Sands MI, Grimes D, Bergman U, Daling J, Mills A: Modern oral contraceptives and cardiovascular disease. Am J Obstet Gynecol 1997;177:707–715.

7. International Federation of Fertility Societies. Consensus conference on combination oral contraceptives and cardiovascular disease Fertil Steril 1999;71(Suppl 3):1S-6S.

8. Inman WHW et al.: Thromboembolic disease and the steroidal content of oral contraceptives: A report to the Committee on Safety of Drugs. Br Med J 1970;2:203–209.

9. Meade TW, Greenberg G, Thompson SF: Progestogens and cardiovascular reactions associated with oral contraceptives and a com-

parison of the safety of 50 and 30 mg oestrogen preparations. Br Med J 1980;280:1157.

10. Beller FK et al.: Effects of oral contraceptives on blood coagulation: A review. Obstet Gynecol Surv 1985;40(7):425–436.

11. Mattson RH, Cramer JA, Caldwell BV, Siconolfi BC: Treatment of seizures with medroxyprogesterone acetate: Preliminary report. Neurology 1984;34:1255–1258.

12. Mol BWJ, Ankum WM, Bossuyt PMM, Van der Veen F: Contraception and the risk of ectopic pregnancy: A meta-analysis. Contraception 1995;52:337–341.

13. Wells JP, Dickey RP, Porter CW: Report of the survey team concerning the decrease in pill acceptors in the Phillipines Family Planning Program, March 22, 1973. American Public Health Association, 1015 18th Street NW, Washington, D.C. 20036.

14. Royal College of General Practitioners Oral Contraceptive Study. Further analysis of mortality in oral contraceptive users. Lancet 1981;1:541.

15. Thomas SHL: Mortality from venous thromboembolism and myocardial infarction in young adults in England and Wales. Lancet 1996;348:402.

16. Dunn Nicholas et al.: Oral contraceptives and myocardial infarction: Results of the MICA casecontrol study. Br Med J 1999;June 12(318):1579–1583.

17. Farley T, Collins J, Schlesselman J: Hormonal contraception and the risk of cardiovascular disease: An international perspective. Contraception 1998;57:211–230.

18. Jick H, Jick SS, Meyers MW, Vasilakis C: Risk of acute myocardial infarction and low-dose combined oral contraceptives. Lancet 1996;347:627–628.

19. Lewis MA, Spitzer WO, Heinemann LAJ, MacRae KD, Bruppacher R, Thorogood M: Third-generation oral contraceptives and risk of myocardial infarction: An international case-control study. BMJ 1996;312:88–90.

20. World Health Organization (WHO) Collaborative Study of Cardiovascular Disease and Steroid Hormone Contraception. Acute myocardial infarction and combined oral contraceptives: Results of an international multicentre case control study. Lancet 1997;349:1202–1209.

21. Wynn V: Effect of duration of low-dose oral contraceptive administration on carbohydrate metabolism. Am J Obstet Gynecol 1982;142:739. 402. Wynn V: Vitamins and oral contraceptive use. Lancet 1975;1:561–564.

22. Khader Y, Rice J, John L, Abueita O. Oral contraceptives use and the risk of myocardial infarction: ameta analysis Contraception 2003;68:11–7.

23. Tanis BC, van den Bosch AAJ, Ke,,eren JM, Cats VM, Helmerhorst FM, Alga A, van der Graaf Y, Rosendaal FR. Oral contraceptives and the risk of myocardial infarction. N Engl J Med 2001; 345:1787–93.

24. Dunn NR, Arscott A, Thorogood M. The relationship between use of oral contraceptives and myocardial infarction in young women with fatal outcome, compared to those who survive: results from the MICA case-control study Contraception 2001;63:65–9.

25. Lewis M, Spitzer WO, Heinemann LAJ, et al.: Lowered risk of dying of heart attack with thirdgeneration contraceptives may offset risk of dying of thromboembolism. Br Med J 1997;315:679–680.

26. Spitzer WO, Lewis MA, Heinemann LAJ, Thorogood M, MacRae KD: Third-generation oral contraceptives and risk of venous thromboembolic disorders: An international case control study. BMJ 1996;312:83–87.

27. Mant Jonathan, Painter Rosemary, Vessey Martin: Risk of myocardial infarction, angina, and stroke in users of oral contraceptives: An updated analysis of a cohort study. Br J Obstet Gynaecol 1998;105:890–896.

28. Dunn NR, Thorogood M, de Caestecker L, Mann RD: Myocardial infarction and oral contraceptives: A retrospective case-control study in England and Scotland (MICA study). Pharmacoepidemiol Drug Safety 1997;6:283–289.

29. Lewis MA, Heinemann LAJ, Spitzer WO, MacRae KD, Bruppacher R: The use of oral contraceptives and the occurrence of acute myocardial infarction in young women. Contraception 1997;56: 129–140.

30. Goldbaum GM et al.: The relative impact of smoking and oral contraceptive use on women in the United States. JAMA 1987;258: 1339.

31. Kloosterboer HJ, Deckers GHJ: Desogestrel: A selective progestogen. Int Proc J 1989;1:26–30.

32. Duffy TJ, Ray R: Oral contraceptive use: Prospective follow-up of women with suspected glucose intolerance. Contraception 1984;30(3): 197–208.

33. Jensen G, Nyboe J, Appleyard M, Schnohr P: Risk factors for acute myocardial infarction in Copenhagen. II: Smoking, alcohol intake, physical activity, obesity, oral contraception, diabetes, lipids, and blood pressure. Eur Heart 1991;12:298–308.

34. TIMI [Thrombosis in Myocardial Infarction] Study Group. The thrombolisis in myocardial infarction (TIMI) trial, Phase I findings. N Engl J Med 1985;312:932–936.

35. Jick Susan S, Myers Marian W, Jick Hershel: Risk of idiopathic cerebral haemorrhage in women on oral contraceptives with differing progestagen components. Lancet 1999;July 24(354):302–303.

36. Lidegaard O, Kreiner S: Cerebral thrombosis and oral contraceptives: A case-control study. Contraception 1998;57:303–314.

37. Longstretch WT, Nelson LM, Koepsell TD, van Belle G: Subarachnoid hemorrhage and hormonal factors in women: A population-based, case control study. Ann Intern Med 1994;121:168–173.

38. Poulter NR et al. and the WHO Collaborative Study of Cardiovascular Disease and Steroid Hormone Contraception: Effect of stroke on different progestagens in low oestrogen dose oral contraceptives. Lancet 1999;July 24(354):301–302.

39. Thorogood M, Mann J, Murphy M, Vessey M: Fatal stroke and use of oral contraceptives: Findings from a case control study. Am J Epidemiol 1992;136:35–45.

40. World Health Organizaton (WHO) Collaborative Study of Cardiovascular Disease and Steroid Hormone Contraception. Hemorrhagic stroke, overall stroke risk, and combined oral contraceptives: Results of an international multicentre case control study. Lancet 1996;348:505–510.

41. World Health Organization (WHO) Collaborative Study of Cardiovascular Disease and Steroid Hormone Contraception. Ischemic stroke and combined oral contraceptives: Results of an international multicentre case control study. Lancet 1996;348:498–505.

42. Petitti DB, Sidney S, Bernstein A, Wolf S, Quesenberry C, Ziel HK: Stroke in users of lowdose oral contraceptives. N Engl J Med 1996;335:8–15.

43. Lidegaard O: Oral contraceptives, pregnancy, and the risk of cerebral thromboembolism: The influence of diabetes, hypertension, migraine, and previous thrombotic disease. Br J Obstet Gynaecol 1995;102:153–159.

44. Lidegaard O: Oral contraception and risk of a cerebral thromboembolic attack: Result of a case control study. British Med Journal 1993;306:956–963.

45. Heinemann Lothar AJ et al.: Thromboembolic stroke in young women: A European case-control study on oral contraceptives. Contraception 1998;57:29–37.

46. Petitti D, Wingerd J: Use of oral contraceptives, cigarette smoking, and risk of subarachnoid hemorrhage. Lancet 1978;2:234–236.

47. Hannaford PC, Croft PR, Kay CR: Oral contraception and stroke: Evidence from the Royal College of General Practitioners' Oral Contraception Study. Stroke 1994;25:935–942.

48. National Institute of Neurological Disorders and Stroke rt-PA Stroke Study Group. Tissue plasminogen activator for acute ischemic stroke. N Engl J Med 1995;333:1581–1587.

49. Farmer R, Preston T: The risk of venous thromboembolism associated with low oestrogen dose oral contraceptives. J Obstet Gynecol 1995;15:195–200.

50. Farmer RDT, Lawrenson RA, Thompson CR, et al.: Population-based study of the risk of venous thromboembolism associated with low-oestrogen dose oral contraceptives. Lancet 1997;349:83–88.

51. Gerstman B, Piper J, Tomita D, Ferguson W, Stadel B, Lundin F: Oral contraceptive dose and the risk of deep venous thromboembolic disease. Am J Epidemiol 1991;133:32–37.

52. Jick H, Jick SS, Gurewich V, Myers MW, Vasilakis C: Risk of ideopathic cardiovascular death and nonfatal venous thromboembolism in women using oral contraceptives with differing progestogen components. Lancet 1995;346:1589–1593.

53. Lidegaard O, Edstrom B, Kreiner S: Oral contraceptives and venous thromboembolism: A case-control study. Contraception 1998;57:291–301.

54. Mills A: Combined oral contraception and the risk of venous thromboembolism. Hum Repro 1997;12:2595–2598.

55. World Health Organization (WHO) Collaborative study on cardiovascular disease and steroid hormone contraception. Venous thromboembolic disease and combined oral contraceptives: Results of international multicentre case control study. Lancet 1995;346:1575–1582.

56. World Health Organization (WHO) Scientific Group on Cardiovascular Disease and Steroid Hormone Contraception. Cardiovascular disease and steroid hormone contraception: A report of a WHO scientific group. WHO technical report series 877. 1997;Geneva.

57. Sparrow MJ: Pregnancies in reliable pill takers. New Zealand Med J 1989;102:575–577.

58. Herings RMC, Urquhart J, Leufkens HGM: Venous thromboembolism among new users of different oral contraceptives. Lancet 1999;July 10(354):127–128.

59. Allaart CF, Poort SR, Rosendaal FR, et al.: Increased risk of venous thrombosis in carriers of hereditary protein C deficiency defect. Lancet 1993;341:134–138.

60. Bloemenkamp KWM, Rosendaal FR, Helmerhorst FM, Buller HR, Vandenbroucke JP: Enhancement by Factor V Leiden mutation

of risk of deep vein thrombosis associated with oral contraceptives containing a third-generation progestagen. Lancet 1995;346: 1593–1596.

61. Rosing J, Trans G, Nicolaes GAF, et al.: Oral contraceptives and venous thrombosis: Different sensitivities to activated protein C in women using second- and third-generation oral contraceptives. Br J Haematol 1997;97:233–238.

62. Vandenbrouke JP, Koster T, Briet E, et al.: Increased risk of venous thrombosis in oral contraceptive users who are carriers of Factor V Leiden mutation. Lancet 1994;344:1453–1457.

63. Jain AK: Mortality risk associated with the use of oral contraceptives. Stud Fam Plann 1977;8:50–54.

64. Suissa S, Blais L, Spitzer WO, Cusson J: Firsttime use of newer oral contraceptives and the risk of venous thromboembolism. Contraception 1997;56:128–132.

65. Vasilakis Catherine, Jick Susan S, Jick Hershel: The risk of venous thromboembolism in users of postcoital contraceptive pills. Contraception 1999;59:79–83.

66. Spitzer WO: The 1995 pill scare revisited: Anatomy of a nonepidemic. Hum Reprod 1997;12:2347–1357.

67. Svensson PJ, Dahlback B: Resistance to activated protein C as a basis for venous thrombosis. New Engl J Med 330:517–522.

68. Allebeck P et al.: Do oral contraceptives reduce the incidence of rheumatoid arthritis? Scand J Rheumatol 1984;13:140.

69. Winkler U: Blood coagulation and oral contraceptives: A critical review. Contraception 1998;57:203–209.

70. Inman WHW, Vessey MP: Investigation of deaths from pulmonary, coronary, and cerebral thrombosis and embolism in women of childbearing age. Br Med J 1968;2:193–199.

71. Rosenberg MJ, Waugh MS, Stevens CM: Smoking and cycle control among oral contraceptive users. Am J Obstet Gynceol 1996; 174:628–632.

72. Royal College of General Practitioners. Oral contraception and thromboembolic disease. J Coll Gen Pract 1967;13:267–279.

73. Royal College of General Practitioners. Oral contraceptives and health: An interim report from the oral contraception study of the Royal College of General Practitioners. New York: Pitman, 1974.

74. Sartwell PE et al.: Thromboembolism and oral contraceptives: An epidemiological case control study. Am J Epidemiol 1969; 90:365–380.

75. Vessey MP, Doll R: Investigation of relation between use of oral contraceptives and thromboembolic disease: A further report. Br Med J 1969;2:651–657.

76. Vessey MP, McPherson K, Yeates D: Mortality in oral contraceptive users. Lancet 1981;1:549.

77. Creinin Mitchell D, Lisman Rachel, Strickler Ronald C: Screening for Factor V Leiden mutation before prescribing combination oral contraceptives. Fertil Steril 1999;October (72)4:646–651.

78. Greene GR, Sartwell PE: Oral contraceptive use in patients with thromboembolism following surgery, trauma or infection. Am J Pub Health 1972;62:680–685.

79. Vessey MP et al.: Postoperative thromboembolism and the use of oral contraceptives. Br Med J 1970;3:123–126.

80. Barter JF et al.: Inferior vena cava thrombosis with oral contraceptives documented by computed tomography. Obstet Gynecol 1983;61(3 Suppl):59S-62S.

81. Hoyle M et al.: Small bowel ischaemia and infarction in young women taking oral contraceptives and progestational agents. Br Med J 1977;64:533.

82. Northmann VJ, Chittinand S, Schuster MN: Reversible mesenteric vascular occlusion associated with oral contraceptives. Am J Digestive Dis 1973;18:361.

83. Weinstein E, Silverman L: Splenic artery thrombosis secondary to oral contraceptive medication: A case report. Milit Med 1982; 147(7):589–590.

84. Jacobs MB: Hepatic infarction related to oral contraceptive use. Arch Intern Med 1984;144(3):642–643.

85. Lewis JH, Tice HL, Zimmerman HJ: Budd-Chiari syndrome associated with oral contraceptive steroids: Review of treatment of 47 cases. Dig Dis Sci 1983;28(8):673–683.

86. Valla D et al.: Risk of hepatic vein thrombosis in relation to recent use of oral contraceptives: A case-control study. Gastroenterology 1986; 90(4):807–811.

87. Zafrani ES, Pinaudeau Y, Dhumeaux D: Drug-induced vascular lesions of the liver. Arch Intern Med 1983;143:495–502.

88. Zafrani ES et al.: Focal hemorrhagic necrosis of the liver. Gastroenterology 1980;79:1295–1299.

89. Dickey RP, Stone SC: Drugs that affect the breast and lactation. Clin Obstet Gynecol 1975;18:2.

90. Blumenstein BA, Douglas MB, Hall WD: Blood pressure changes and oral contraceptive use: A study of 2,676 black women in the southeastern United States. Am J Epidemiol 1980;112: 539–552.

91. Lubianca JN, Faccin CS, Fuchs FD. Oral contraceptives: a risk factor for uncontrolled blood pressure among hypertensive women. Contraception 2003;67:19–24.

92. Cook NR et al.: Regression analysis of changes in blood pressure with oral contraceptive use. Am J Epidemiol 1985;121(4): 530–540.

93. Royal College of General Practitioners Oral Contraceptive Study. Effect on hypertension and benign breast disease of progestogen component in combined oral contraceptives. Lancet 1977;1:624.

SECTION 27: ENDOCRINE AND METABOLIC SYSTEMS

DIABETES MELLITUS

Clinical Information

Women who require insulin prior to OC use have not been reported to experience worsening of their conditions or increased needs for insulin while taking OCs. There is no evidence that OC use increases renal or cardiovascular complications in insulin-dependent diabetics (1, 2).

Women who develop gestational diabetes (Class A) during pregnancy and those with strong family histories of diabetes in parents or siblings have the greatest potential for having altered glucose tolerance tests (GTTs) during OC use (3, 4). Deterioration in the GTT is progressive and is accompanied by a persistent elevation of insulin levels in relation to serum glucose (hyperinsulinemia) (5, 6).

Hyperinsulinemia does not seem to occur in women taking low-dose OCs containing 0.4 or 0.5 mg norethindrone combined with 35 mcg EE or triphasic OCs containing norethindrone (7, 8, 9).

Carbohydrate metabolism appears to be less affected by the new progestins desogestrel, gestodene, and norgestimate than by second-generation progestins (10, 11). Progestin implants have not been shown to alter glucose levels in healthy women and cause only a slight increase in fasting glucose levels (12).

Symptoms of hypoglycemia (weakness and irritability two to four hours after a high-glucose meal) occur in some OC users. Hypoglycemia is related to progestin type and dose.

OCs have been shown to impair oral glucose tolerance (13). Glucose tolerance changes are reversible in most patients after they discontinue OC use, but some cases of glucose intolerance progression to insulin dependence have been reported (14).

Causal Factors

The effects of combination OCs on carbohydrate metabolism are complex (15, 16, 17, 18, 19). Utilization of glucose usually deteriorates with a compensatory increase in insulin secretion during OC use. Progestins cause a decrease and estrogens an increase in the number of insulin receptors on the cell membrane. Progestins increase insulin secretion and create insulin resistance. Estrogen causes glucose intolerance with impaired insulin secretion. Estrogens may also slow the uptake of glucose from the gastrointestinal tract.

Management

Due to the high incidence of maternal and fetal morbidity and mortality in women with insulin-dependent diabetes (IDD) should not be denied the benefits of OCs if other methods of contraception are unreliable or unacceptable (20, 21, 22, 23). Women at high risk for diabetes should initially be given OCs with progestin activities equal to or less than 0.5 mg norethindrone.

Prior to starting OCs and annually during OC use, patients at risk for IDD should have fasting blood sugar determinations or two-hour postprandial sugar tests, although full GTTs are preferable. These tests should be repeated during the second or third cycle of OC use. If a marked change is observed in glucose tolerance (significantly higher serum glucose levels), these patients should stop OC use. Once their glucose levels return to normal, patients may be switched to OCs with lower estrogen/progesterone activities and the pills restarted. If glucose levels again become abnormal, patients should permanently discontinue OC use and use alternative contraceptive methods. Oral hypoglycemic medications should not be used in order that OCs may be continued.

Diabetic OC users are at increased risk of cardiovascular disease. Clinicians may wish to counsel these patients who have achieved their desired family size about permanent contraception (sterilization). Patients experiencing symptoms of hypoglycemia should be switched to OCs with lower progestational and androgenic or greater estrogenic activities. Low-

27.

carbohydrate/high-protein diet modification should also be prescribed.

ADRENAL CHANGES

Clinical Information

Adrenal changes during OC use include a slight rise in free cortisol and protein-bound serum cortisol levels.

After OCs are stopped, corticosteroid sex-binding globulin (CSBG)-bound cortisol levels may remain elevated and free progesterone levels may be decreased until CSBG levels return to normal. The first cycles after OCs are stopped and even early pregnancy may be associated with progesterone deficiency. Steroid-sensitive women may experience a worsening of their conditions when they discontinue OCs.

In one study, dehydroeplandrosterone (DHEAS) levels decreased 30 to 40% in women using OCs containing 0.4 to 1 mg norethindrone but not in women using OCs containing 0.15 mg LNG (24).

Causal Factors

OCs cause an increase in CSBG (transcortin) because of the estrogen component. High doses of estrogens alter the hepatic metabolism of corticosteroids.

Progesterone and progestins derived from progesterone are bound to CSBG but not to sex steroid-binding globulin (SSBG); those derived from 19-nor-testosterone are not bound to CSBG.

Management

No treatment is required for mild elevations in serum cortisol during OC use. The slight elevation of free cortisol may result in relief of arthritis and other inflammatory conditions.

THYROID CHANGES

Clinical Information

OCs cause increased serum levels of bound thyroxin (T4), but unbound T4 and thyroid-stimulating hormone

(TSH) are unchanged. A mild clinical hypothyroid state may be hidden by apparently normal T4 levels while OCs are being used and for several months after they are discontinued. No association between thyroid disease and OC use per se was found by either the RCGP study (25) or the Walnut Creek study (26).

Thyroid nodules and thyroid neoplasia are not related to OC use but may be detected for the first time in OC users because of the relatively higher incidence in the reproductive age group. The incidence of malignancy in thyroid nodules is high; 20% of active (hot) nodules and 70% of inactive (cold) nodules are malignant in women of reproductive age.

Women with undiagnosed hyperthyroidism or hypothyroidism may experience decreased or increased symptoms, respectively, from OCs.

Causal Factors

Changes in bound T4 are due to estrogen, which causes an increase in thyroid-binding globulin (TBG). There may be no change in free T4 concentration.

Management

The thyroid gland should be palpated and deep tendon reflexes checked before OCs are started, and annually thereafter. All patients with thyroid nodules require further evaluation, including radioactive iodine scans. OCs may be used safely by most women with treated thyroid disorders (27).

References for Section 27: Endocrine and Metabolic Systems

1. Jackson WE: Oral contraceptives and renal and retinal complications in young women with insulindependent diabetes meliitus. JAMA 1994;271:1099–1102.
2. Peterson KR, Skouby SO, Sidelmann J, Molsted- Pederson L, Jesperson J: Effects of contraceptive steroids on cardiovascular risk factors in women with insulin-dependent diabetes mellitus. Am J Obstet Gynecol 1994;171:400–405.
3. Kung AW, Ma JT, Wong VC, et al.: Glucose and lipid metabolism with triphasic oral contraceptives in women with history of gestational diabetes. Contraception 1987;35:257–269.

4. Szabo AG, Cole HS, Grimaldi RD: Glucose tolerance in gestational diabetic women during and after treatment with the combination type oral contraceptives. N Engl J Med 1970;282:646.

5. Shoupe D: Effects of oral contraceptives on the borderline NIDD patient. Int J Fertil 1991;36:80–86.

6. Shoupe D, Kjos S: Effects of oral contraceptives on the borderline NIDD patient. Int J Fertil 1988;33:27–34.

7. Wynn V: Effect of duration of low-dose oral contraceptive administration on carbohydrate metabolism. Am J Obstet Gynecol 1982;142:739.

8. Wynn V et al.: Comparison of effects of different combined oral contraceptive formulations on carbohydrate and lipid metabolism. Lancet 1979;1:1045–1049.

9. Wynn V et al.: Effects of oral contraceptives on carbohydrate metabolism. J Reprod Med 1986;31(9 Suppl):892–897.

10. Luyckx AS et al.: Carbohydrate metabolism in women who used oral contraceptives containing LNG or desogestrel: A six-month prospective study. Fertil Steril 1986;45(5):635–642.

11. Speroff L, DeCherney A, et al.: Evaluation of a new generation of oral contraceptives. Obstet Gynecol 1993;81:1034–1047.

12. Skouby SO, Molsted-Pedersen L, Kuhl C, Bennet P: Oral contraceptives in diabetic women: Metabolic effects of four compounds with different estrogen/progestogen profiles. Fertil Steril 1986;46:858–864.

13. Vessey MP, Doll R: Investigation of relation between use of oral contraceptives and thromboembolic disease. Br Med J 1968;2:199–205.

14. Duffy TJ, Ray R: Oral contraceptive use: Prospective follow-up of women with suspected glucose intolerance. Contraception 1984;30(3): 197–208.

15. Berenson AB, Weimann CM, Rickerr VI, McCombs SL: Contraceptive outcome among adolescents prescribed Norplant® implants vs oral contraceptives after one year of use. Am J Obstet Gynecol 1997;176:586–592.

16. De Pirro R et al.: Changes in insulin receptors during oral contraception. J Clin Endo Metab 1981;52:29.

17. Godsland IF, Walton C, Felton C, Proudler A, Patel A: Insulin resistance, secretion, metabolism in users of oral contraceptives. J Clin Endocrinol Metab 1991;74:64–70.

18. Kalkoff RW: Effect of oral contraceptive agents and sex steroids on carbohydrate metabolism. Ann Rev Med 1972;23:429–438.

19. Wynn V, Doar JWH, Mills GL: Some effects of oral contraceptives on serum lipid and lipoprotein levels. Lancet 1966;2:720–723.

20. Fuller JH et al.: Coronary heart disease risk and impaired glucose tolerance: The Whitehall study. Lancet 1980;1:1373.

21. Gaspard UJ, Lefebvre PJ: Clinical aspects of the relationship between oral contraceptive, abnormalities in carbohydrate metabolism, and the development of cardiovascular disease. Am J Obstet Gynecol 1990;163:334–343.

22. Jensen G, Nyboe J, Appleyard M, Schnohr P: Risk factors for acute myocardial infarction in Copenhagen. II: Smoking, alcohol intake, physical activity, obesity, oral contraception, diabetes, lipids, and blood pressure. Eur Heart 1991;12:298–308.

23. Mestman JH, Schmidt-Sarosi C: Diabetes mellitus and fertility control: Contraception management issues. Am J Obstet Gynecol 1993;168:2012–1020.

24. Klove KL, Roy S, Lobo RA: The effect of different contraceptive treatments on the serum concentration of dehydroepiandrosterone sulfate. Contraception 1984;29(4):319–324.

25. Royal College of General Practitioners. Oral contraceptives and health: An interim report from the oral contraception study of the Royal College of General Practitioners. New York: Pitman, 1974.

26. Ramcharan S, Pellegrin FA, Ray RM, Hsu JP: The Walnut Creek Contraceptive Drug Study: A prospective study of the side effects of oral contraceptives. J Reprod Med 1980;25:345–372.

27. Loriaux L, Wild RA: Contraceptive choices for women with endocrine disorders. Am J Obstet Gynecol 1993;168:2021–2026.

SECTION 28:
GASTROINTESTINAL SYSTEM

NAUSEA/VOMITING

Clinical Information

Nausea and vomiting are most severe during the first cycles of OC use and usually disappear with time. Symptoms occur more often in women who have experienced marked nausea during pregnancy (1). Nausea that occurs several hours after meals may be due to hypoglycemia. Vomiting and diarrhea were reported by 34% of women with "pill failure" who had not missed taking their OCs (2).

Causal Factors

Nausea similar to morning sickness of early pregnancy is common in OC users and is related to the estrogen dose. In a placebo-controlled, double-blind, cross-over study, nausea and vomiting were related to the estrogen content of OCs (3). Hypoglycemia is related to the progestin component of OCs. Most nausea is caused by gastrointestinal disease and not by OC use.

Management

Patients may relieve nausea by taking their OCs with food or at bedtime.

If symptoms persist after the third cycle of OC use or are unusually severe, such patients should be switched to OCs with less estrogenic activities and advised to follow diets low in carbohydrates.

Symptoms of hypoglycemia should be relieved by switching patients to OCs with less progestational activities.

ABDOMINAL BLOATING

Clinical Information

Bloating or swelling of the lower abdomen is common in women having regular ovulatory cycles and is part of the premenstrual complex.

Causal Factors

Premenstrual fluid retention in women not taking OCs is due to the rebound sodium and water retention due to a decrease in progesterone secretion from the aging corpus luteum (4, 5). Progesterone enhances sodium and water excretion, possibly by blocking aldosterone action, while estrogen and androgen cause sodium and water retention. The progestin component of OCs derived from 19-nor-testosterone does not cause sodium and water excretion as progesterone does but may instead cause fluid retention due to the androgenic activity of either the progestin or estrogen component (6).

Abdominal bloating during the period that active OCs are taken may also be caused by a reduction in bowel peristalsis due to the smooth muscle relaxing effect of progestin.

Management

Patients may be switched to OCs with lower estrogenic activities if other fluid retention symptoms are present or to OCs with lower progestational activities if symptoms of progestin and/or androgen excess are present (see Table 6).

28.

ABDOMINAL PAIN

Clinical Information

Abdominal pain may present as abdominal cramping, epigastric distress, or gastritis. Gastritis due to OCs may appear in the first cycle of OC use and with the first OCs in subsequent cycles. This should lessen with continued use (6).

Acute gastritis unrelated to OC use may occur at any time.

Very severe pain may be the result of thrombosis of the mesenteric artery (6, 7, 8) or to other diseases unrelated to OC use (see Section 26).

Causal Factors

Women with nutritionally limited diets frequently complain of:

- Epigastric distress
- Stomach pain
- Abdominal cramps.

Intestinal flu (gastric influenza) is reported almost twice as often (1.89 times) in OC users as in nonusers (9).

Management
OC users may prevent gastritis by taking their pills with food and by using common antacid preparations or by switching to pills with lower estrogen and progestin contents.

DUODENAL AND GASTRIC ULCERS

Duodenal ulcers are 6 to 12 times less common in women than in men. The incidence of duodenal ulcers is further reduced by pregnancy and is decreased by 40% in OC users (9). The reduced incidence is related to the progestin dose. There is no difference in the incidence of gastric ulcers between OC users and nonusers.

ULCERATIVE COLITIS AND REGIONAL ENTERITIS

The incidence of ulcerative colitis was increased twofold and regional enteritis by 40% in OC users in one study (9). Other studies found similar or higher incidences in OC users (10, 11, 12, 13). In a study of hospitalized patients, the risk of regional enteritis was increased eight times in women who used OCs for five years or longer.

The incidence of Crohn's disease appears to increase with years of OC use, but returns to normal within four years after discontinuing OCs.

Women who experience bloody diarrhea for the first time while taking OCs should discontinue use.

Women with ulcerative colitis and regional enteritis should be observed closely and OCs stopped if increasing severity of disease or frequency of attacks occurs.

ORAL LESIONS

Several surveys and case reports indicate an increased incidence of gingivitis in OC users. One large survey found an increase of about 30% in periapical abscess, chronic gingivitis, and mouth ulcers, conditions unrelated to OC dose (9). This rate increase may have been the result of over-reporting.

Hyperplasia of the gums (gingivitis) also occurs more frequently in pregnant women, but the cause is unknown. Mouth ulcers due to the herpes simplex virus are more common in OC users.

Salivary calculi are increased 76% in OC users, but the total incidence is small (less than 0.3 per 1,000 women per years of use) (9).

If these conditions recur, patients may be switched to OCs with reduced doses of estrogen and progestin.

OCs do not cause thrush (14).

Female sex steroids may affect wound healing after tooth extraction (15).

References for Section 28: Gastrointestinal System

1. Dickey RP, Chihal HJW, Peppler R: Potency of three new low-estrogen pills. Am J Obstet Gynecol 1976;125:976–979.
2. Sparrow MJ: Pill method failures. New Zealand Med J 1987;100:102–105.
3. Goldzieher Joseph W et al.: A placebo-controlled, double-blind, cross-over investigation of the side effects attributed to oral contraceptives. Fertil Steril 1971;22:609–623.
4. Dickey RP: Oral contraceptives: Basic considerations. In: Human Reproduction, Conception, and Contraception. 2nd ed. Hafez ESE (ed.) Hagerstown, PA: Harper and Row, 1978.
5. Dickey RP: The pill: Physiology, pharmacology, and clinical use. In: Seminar in Family Planning, 1st ed. Isenman AW, Knox EG, Tyrer L (eds.) American College of Obstetrics and Gynecology, 1972. 2nd ed., 1974.
6. Dickey RP, Dorr CH II: Oral contraceptives: Selection of the proper pill. Obstet Gynecol 1969;33:273.
7. Barter JF et al.: Inferior vena cava thrombosis with oral contraceptives documented by computed tomography. Obstet Gynecol 1983;61(3 Suppl):59S-62S.

8. Northmann VJ, Chittinand S, Schuster MN: Reversible mesenteric vascular occlusion associated with oral contraceptives. Am J Digestive Dis 1973;18:361.

9. Royal College of General Practitioners. Oral contraceptives and health: Aninterim report from the oral contraception study of the Royal College of General Practitioners. New York: Pitman, 1974.

10. Entrican JH, Sircus W: Chronic inflammatory bowel disease, cigarette smoking, and use of oral contraceptives (letter). Br Med J (Clin Res) 1986;292(6533):1464.

11. Lesko SM et al.: Evidence for an increased risk of Crohn's disease in oral contraceptive users. Gastroenterology 1985;89(5):1046–1049.

12. Rhodes JM et al.: Colonic Crohn's disease and use of oral contraception. Br Med J (Clin Res) 1984;288(6417):595–596.

13. Vessey MP et al.: Chronic inflammatory bowel disease, cigarette smoking, and use of oral contraceptives: Findings in a large cohort study of women of childbearing age. Br Med J (Clin Res) 1986;292(6528):1101–1103.

14. Davidson F et al.: The pill does not cause thrush. Br J Obstet Gynaecol 1985;92(12):1265–1266.

15. Gansicke A, Gansicke W, Klammt J: Effect of female sex hormones on the incidence of disordered wound healing following tooth extraction. Zahn Mund Kieferheilkd 1986;74(2):131–137.

NOTES

SECTION 29: HEPATIC SYSTEM

CHOLECYSTITIS/CHOLELITHIASIS

Clinical Information

Cholecystitis (inflammation) or cholelithiasis (gall-stones) may be increased in OC users (1, 2, 3, 4, 5).

The incidence of surgically confirmed cholecystitis and cholelithiasis is twice as high in OC users as in nonusers in the U.S.; the same relationship was not found in England. A retrospective study in the U.S. found an annual attack rate of 158 per 100,000 OC users; a British prospective study found a rate of 68 per 100,000 OC users, which was not significantly different from the rate found for nonusers.

Two studies from Australia and the U.S. found that the risk of developing gallstones with OC use was highest in young women, and was low or none existent in older women. In one study, an increased risk appeared after two years of OC use and doubled after four or five years of use. In another study, an increased risk was apparent between 6 and 12 months of use.

Obstructive jaundice due to cholelithiasis occurs only rarely and is accompanied by other symptoms.

There are no data to suggest that prior gallbladder disease is a contraindication to OC use.

Some studies have found an increased risk of surgically confirmed gallbladder disease in users of estrogens. Sonographic studies have found no effect of OCs on gallbladder function.

Causal Factors

Reduced cholesterol excretion, possibly caused by progestins, results in cholesterol precipitation in the gall-bladder, so that gallstones are formed.

Management

The onset of cholecystitis and cholelithiasis is characterized by acute abdominal pain. Women with abdominal pain require complete medical evaluation. Other conditions with similar symptoms may be fatal.

The risk of cholecystitis and cholelithiasis and the incidence of repeated attacks of these diseases may be reduced by use of low progestin-dose OCs.

CHOLESTATIC JAUNDICE AND PRURITUS

Clinical Information
Causes of cholestatic jaundice include:
- Hepatocanalicular jaundice
- Cholangiolitic hepatitis
- Obstructive jaundice.

Cholestatic jaundice in OC users is rare, although some individuals and ethnic groups (e.g., Scandinavians and Chileans) appear to be more susceptible. Approximately 50% of OC jaundice occurs during the first cycle of OC use and 90% during the first six cycles (3).

Symptoms of jaundice and pruritus are the cardinal signs of cholestatic jaundice.

After OCs are discontinued, tests of liver function and hepatic histology become normal and jaundice usually disappears completely within two to three months.

If jaundice of pregnancy occurs, it is more likely to recur in subsequent pregnancies.

Causal Factors
Cholestatic jaundice may be the sequel of infectious hepatitis or it may follow use of:
- Methyltestosterone or other androgens
- Sulfonamides
- Thiouracil
- Triacetyloleandomycin (TAO).

Both the estrogen and progestin components of OCs can cause liver dysfunction. Synthesis and/or release of gamma-glutamyl transpeptidase appear to be decreased during OC use and during the second half of pregnancy. The use of OCs with TAO and perhaps other drugs associated with cholestatic jaundice is additive and possibly synergistic (6). Severe alcoholic cirrhosis but not primary biliary cirrhosis affects the metabolism of medroxyprogesterone acetate (MPA) (7). The effect on the metabolism of other contraceptive steroids is uncertain.

Management

If jaundice occurs, OCs should be stopped until its cause can be determined. If an etiology other than OC use can be determined, OCs may be restarted after liver function tests return to normal or three months after clinical symptoms disappear. If symptoms recur, OCs should be permanently discontinued.

HEPATOMA AND MALIGNANT LIVER TUMOR

Clinical Information

Liver changes associated with OC use may include:
- Hepatoma (benign adenoma)
- Cholangiocarcinoma
- Hepatocellular carcinoma.

Women who use OCs for five years or longer appear to have an increased risk of developing benign or malignant liver neoplasms (8, 9, 10, 11, 12, 13, 14, 15, 16, 17). There is little or no increased risk for short-term use; nor is there an increase in cholangiocarcinoma.

A 1995 meta-analysis estimated the risk of liver cancer in nonusers of OCs from ages 20 to 54 to be 20 per 100,000 women. For women who used OCs for eight years, an estimated additional 41 liver cancers developed (18). However, population-based data do not support evidence of a measurable effect of OCs on primary liver cancer (19).

Although they are benign, hepatic adenomas may rupture and cause death through intra-abdominal hemorrhage. This has been reported in short- as well as long-term OC users. Two studies relate risk to duration of use, the risk being much greater after four or more years of OC use. A 2002 case control study estimated that every use of OCs increased the incidence of focal nodular hyperplasia of the liver 2.8 fold, and that use of OCs for > 3 years increased the incidence 4.5 fold (20). While hepatic adenoma is a rare lesion, it should be considered in women with abdominal pain, tenderness, or mass.

Causal Factors

It has been proposed that estrogens are important in the genesis of liver tumors by impairing biliary secretions and causing decreased blood flow. However, testosterone and androgenic drugs are reported to increase the incidence of hepatoma in both men and women. Infection from the hepatitis B virus is strongly associated with hepatocellular carcinoma.

Management

All OC users should have the edge of the liver palpated at their annual or semi-annual examinations. This becomes more important after OCs have been taken for several years. If a liver mass is discovered, OCs must be stopped immediately.

Benign liver tumors regress in size after OCs are stopped, so that surgery may not be necessary.

Women with histories of the hepatitis B virus should be advised not to use steroidal contraception due to the increased risk of hepatocellular carcinoma.

References for Section 29: Hepatic and Biliary Systems

1. Boston Collaborative Drug Surveillance Program. Oral contraceptives and venous thromboembolic disease, surgically-confirmed gallbladder disease, and breast tumors. Lancet 1973;1:1399–1404.
2. Braverman DZ et al.: Effects of pregnancy and contraceptive steroids on gallbladder function. New Engl J Med 1980;302:362.
3. Royal College of General Practitioners. Oral contraceptives and health: An interim report from the oral contraception study of the Royal College of General Practitioners. New York: Pitman, 1974.

221

4. Scragg RK, McMichael AJ, Seamark RF: Oral contraceptives, pregnancy, and endogenous oestrogen in gallstone disease: A case control study. Br Med J (Clin Res) 1984;288(6433): 1795–1799.

5. Strom BL et al.: Oral contraceptives and other risk factors for gallbladder disease. Clin Pharmacol Ther 1986;39(3):335–341.

6. Haber I, Hubens H: Cholestatic jaundice after triacetyloleandomycin and oral contraceptives. Acta Gastro-Enterol Belgica 1980;43:475.

7. Rautio A: Liver function and medroxyprogesterone acetate elimination in man. Biomed and Pharmacother 1984;38:199.

8. Baum J et al.: Possible association between benign hepatomas and oral contraceptives. Lancet 1973;2:926–929.

9. Federal Drug Administration Drug Bulletin. April 1990;5.

10. Forman D, Vincent TJ, Doll R: Cancer of the liver and the use of oral contraceptives. Br Med J 1986;292(6532):1357–1361.

11. Huggins GR, Guintoli RL: Oral contraceptives and neoplasia. Fertil Steril 1979;32:1.

12. Mays ET et al.: Hepatic changes in young women ingesting contraceptive steroids: Hepatic hemorrhage and primary hepatic tumors. JAMA 1976;235:730–732.

13. Neuberger J et al.: Oral contraceptive-associated liver tumors: Occurrence of malignancy and difficulties in diagnosis. Lancet 1980;1:273.

14. Neuberger J et al.: Oral contraceptives and hepatocellular carcinoma. Br Med J 1986;292:1355–1357.

15. Newton J et al.: Oral contraceptives and hepatocellular carcinoma. Br Med J (Clin Res) 1986;292:1392.

16. Nissen ED, Kent DR, Nissen SE: Etiologic factors in the pathogenesis of liver tumors associated with oral contraceptives. Am J Obstet Gynecol 1977;127:61.

17. Rooks JB et al.: Epidemiology of hepatocellular adenoma: The role of oral contraceptive use. JAMA 1979;242(7):644–648.

18. Schlesselman JJ: Net effect of oral contraceptive use on the risk of cancer in women in the United States. Obstet Gynecol 1995; 85:793–801.

19. Waetjen LE, Grimes DA: Oral contraceptives and primary liver cancer: Temporal trends in three countries. Obstet Gynecol 1996;88:945–949.

20. Scalori A, Tavani A, Gallus S, La Vecchia C, Colombo M. Oral contraceptives and the risk of focal nodular hyperplasia of the liver: A case control study. Am J Obstet Gynecol 2002;186:195–7.

NOTES

SECTION 30: RESPIRATORY AND URINARY SYSTEMS

RESPIRATORY INFECTIONS

Clinical Information

Acute and chronic respiratory infections appear to be increased for OC users, though the increase may be due to over reporting (1).

OC users also have an increased incidence of:
- Acute nasopharyngitis
- Chronic nasopharyngitis
- Laryngitis
- Tracheitis
- Chronic sinusitis
- Upper respiratory infection
- Acute and chronic bronchitis
- Pneumonia.

Causal Factors

Increased nasal congestion during pregnancy is due to edema and the increased vascularity of mucus membranes caused by estrogen.

Progesterone is known to be immunosuppressive (2, 3).

Management

If respiratory infections recur, patients should discontinue OC use or use OCs with reduced steroid contents.

CHEST PAIN/SHORTNESS OF BREATH

Clinical Information

A twofold increase in pleurisy was found in OC users in a Royal College of General Practitioners (RCGP) study (1).

The possibility of pulmonary embolus should be suspected if chest pain is sudden in onset (see Section 26).

Management

Due to the potentially extreme seriousness of chest pain and shortness of breath, a patient with these symptoms should discontinue OCs and see a physician.

CYSTIC FIBROSIS

Clinical Information

A prospective study of 10 adolescent and young adult OC users with moderate to severe lung disease due to cystic fibrosis found no significant deterioration in clinical status or pulmonary function (4).

URINARY PROBLEMS

Clinical Information

Cystitis and pyelonephritis occur significantly more often in OC users (1).

Lack of estrogenic effects in menopausal women is known to be associated with:

- Uterine and bladder descensus
- Cystocele
- Stress incontinence.

Causal Factors

Progesterone causes dilatation of ureters during pregnancy and may have a similar effect in OC users.

Estrogens cause hypersensitivity of the bladder and increase urinary frequency and urgency.

Management

Cystitis is usually unrelated to OC use. If cystitis should occur more frequently after OCs are started, or if symptoms similar to cystitis occur without bacteria being found in the urine, patients should be switched to OCs with lower estrogenic activities.

If loss of urine occurs and pelvic examination reveals uterine descensus that was not present before use of an OC, a patient should be switched to an OC with higher estrogenic activity.

References for Section 30: Respiratory and Urinary Systems

1. Royal College of General Practitioners. Oral contraceptives and health: An interim report from the oral contraception study of the Royal College of General Practitioners. New York: Pitman, 1974.

2. Baker DA, Thomas J: The effect of low-dose oral contraceptives on the initial immune response to infection. Contraception 1984;29(6):519–525.

3. Munroe JS: Progesterone as immunosuppressive agents. J Reticuloendothelial Soc 1971;9:361.

4. Fitzpatrick SB et al.: Use of oral contraceptives in women with cystic fibrosis. Chest 1984;86(6): 863–867.

NOTES

SECTION 31:
NEUROSENSORY SYSTEM

Sensory/nervous system symptoms are often difficult to assess. Although many of these symptoms are unrelated to OC use, some that appear after OCs are started are of a potentially serious nature and require immediate attention.

HEADACHE

Headaches are among the most common patient complaints regardless of OC use (1, 2). They may be a manifestation of body conditions or disease processes. Most occur in the absence of organic pathological conditions, but some may be associated with serious illness.

Tension Headaches
Tension headaches are commonly characterized as:
* Gradually increasing in intensity
* Nonthrobbing
* Occurring bilaterally in the back of the head and neck
* Occasionally occurring bilaterally at the temples.

Tension headaches are common occurrences. Most are benign and unrelated to OC use.

Headaches Due to Fluid Retention
Fluid retention headaches are associated with:
* Edema of the legs
* Bloating
* Breast tenderness
* Short-term weight gain.

Fluid retention headaches and vascular spasm (migraine) may be related to OC use. Both types are believed to be due to estrogen.

Migrane or Vascular Headaches
Migraine or vascular headaches are characterized as:

228

- Occurring unilaterally
- Progressive in intensity
- Throbbing at their height
- Numbness of an arm or leg
- Sometimes associated with a transient prodrome of:
  - Nausea
  - Dizziness
  - Scintillating scotoma (flashing lights).

In rare cases, increased headaches are a warning sign of hypertension.

In a placebo-controlled, double-blind, cross-over study, headaches that occurred in the first cycle of OC use only were related to high estrogen levels (3).

One study found migraine headaches more severe but not more frequent in OC users. It also found headaches were concentrated in pill-free days and the first days of a new pill cycle (4).

As many as one-third of migraine patients note improvement in their conditions when using OCs.

Ischemic stroke seems to be more common in OC users who first experience migraines while taking OCs than in women who have migraines before using OCs (4).

Management

OC use may be an appropriate choice of contraception for women with pre-existing migraine that does not worsen while taking OCs. However, such women should be monitored closely for an increase in severity or frequency of headaches.

Women who first experience migraine or focal neurological symptoms while taking OCs or who note worsening of pre-existing headaches should stop OC use immediately and substitute with other methods of contraception.

If headaches are clearly associated with fluid excess, patients can be switched to OCs with lower estrogenic activities (see Table 6). If headaches persist after switching OCs, patients should discontinue OCs and use alternative contraceptive methods.

DIZZINESS

Clinical Information

Dizziness includes syncope, vertigo, faint feeling, and lightheadedness.

Dizziness may occur in association with fluid retention and usually disappears after the third cycle of OC use. It may also be due to low blood pressure (hypotension) or severe anemia.

Dizziness that occurs two to four hours after a meal that has a high sugar content may be due to hypoglycemia.

Causal Factors

Although its exact etiology is unknown, dizziness is common in early pregnancy and may be related to estrogen.

Symptoms of hypoglycemia are believed to be due to the progestin component of OCs (see Section 28).

Management

If symptoms persist after the third cycle of OC use, patients may be switched to OCs with lower estrogenic activities. If no relief occurs, other causes of dizziness should be explored.

If symptoms are believed to be due to hypoglycemia, patients should be switched to OCs with lower progestational activities and advised to eat low-carbohydrate diets.

HOT FLUSHES/HOT FLASHES/ HOT FEELINGS

Clinical Information

Hot flushes are uncommon in OC users because even OCs with less than 50 mcg estrogen have estrogenic activities equal to or greater than is used for menopausal hormone replacement.

Hot flushes occurring during the seven days that active OCs are not taken may signal that a woman has reached menopause and no longer needs OCs.

These symptoms are frequent complaints of women in countries that have warm climates.

Causal Factors

Some hot flushes or hot feelings experienced by OC users may be due to the thermogenic effect of progestin. The temperature increase caused by progestins is no greater than that occurring during pregnancy and is not serious or harmful.

Hot flushes during menopause are a vascular effect due to low estrogen or high luteinizing hormone levels.

Localized heat in an extremity may be due to thrombosis (see Section 26).

Management

If hot flushes occur during OC use, patients may be switched to OCs with higher estrogenic or lower progestational activity.

If hot flushes occur during the seven days when active OCs are not taken and patients are near menopause, OCs may be discontinued and other contraceptive methods used for a six-month period. If no menses occur during this time, the woman is probably menopausal and contraceptive efforts may be discontinued.

NUMBNESS OR TINGLING OF EXTREMITIES

Clinical Information

Numbness or tingling of extremities has been described as:

- A pins and needles feeling
- Unilateral or bilateral paralysis
- Weakness of an extremity.

Symptoms of numbness or tingling are usually transient and are relieved after OC use is discontinued.

Unilateral weakness or paralysis occurs preceding migraine attack. The risk of stroke is increased in women with unilateral symptoms.

Causal Factors

These symptoms may signify cerebral vascular spasm if they are unilateral and involve both upper and lower extremities. If bilateral, symptoms may be due to simple fluid retention.

Management

If unilateral symptoms occur, OCs must be discontinued.

Bilateral symptoms of a mild nature may be managed by switching patients to OCs with lower estrogenic activities. If bilateral symptoms persist, OCs should be permanently discontinued.

VISION CHANGES

Clinical Information

Vision changes may include:
- Blurring of vision
- Scintillating scotoma
- Diplopia
- Papilledema
- Difficulty with refraction of lens; this effect is due to swelling secondary to estrogen as often occurs during pregnancy and is not serious
- Proptosis
- Sudden diminished vision
- Sudden loss of vision.

The visual symptoms listed below should be regarded as serious, and OC use should be stopped immediately if they occur. These symptoms may be related to OC use (as have reported neuroocular lesions, such as optic neuritis and retinal artery thrombosis).

Visual symptoms due to vascular spasm that may precede stroke include:
- Scintillating scotoma
- Proptosis

- Sudden diminished vision
- Transient loss of sight.

Management

If unilateral symptoms occur, OCs must be discontinued.

Bilateral symptoms of a mild nature may be managed by switching patients to OCs with lower estrogenic activities. If bilateral symptoms persist, OCs should be permanently discontinued.

HEARING CHANGES

Hearing changes are not believed to be due to OC use. Reduction of ear wax is the only known effect of OCs on hearing, and this is believed to be due to an estrogenic effect of reducing sebum secretion (2). Otosclerosis is unrelated to OC use (5).

SENSE OF SMELL

The sense of smell is not known to be affected by OC use.

SENSE OF TASTE

Taste is sometimes reported to be affected by OC use. Some OC users and some pregnant women report an unpleasant sweet taste in the mouth. OC users may have increased incidences of:
- Salivary calculi
- Gingivitis
- Mouth ulcers (2).

References for Section 31: Neurosensory System

1. Nattero G: Menstrual headache. Adv Neurol 1982;33:215–226.
2. Royal College of General Practitioners. Oral contraceptives and health: An interim report from the oral contraception study of the Royal College of General Practitioners. New York: Pitman, 1974.

3. Goldzieher Joseph W et al.: A placebo-controlled, double-blind, cross-over investigation of the side effects attributed to oral contraceptives. Fertil Steril 1971;22:609–623.

4. Mattson RH, Rebar RW: Contraceptive methods for women with neurologic disorders. Am J Obstet Gynecol 1993;168:2027–2032.

5. Bausch J: Effects and side effects of hormonal contraceptives in the region of the nose, throat, and ear. HNO 1983; (112):409–414.

NOTES

SECTION 32:
NEUROPSYCHOLOGICAL SYSTEM

DEPRESSION

Clinical Information

Depression may be increased in OC users (1).

Depression is a condition marked by:

- Apathy
- Listlessness
- Loss of appetite
- Insomnia
- Restlessness
- Tiredness
- Fatigue
- Sleepiness.

Causal Factors

Symptoms of tiredness and sleepiness in OC users may be due to the progestin component and are similar to symptoms due to increased progesterone in mid- and late-pregnancy.

Similar symptoms may also occur due to low blood sugar (hypoglycemia) or hypothyroidism. Clinicians should investigate these conditions before they switch patients to OCs with different progestin doses.

Chronic tiredness may also be the result of:

- Chronic poor health
- Malnutrition caused by inadequate or "fad" diets
- Severe anemia
- Vitamin B_6 (pyridoxine) deficiency.

Management

Women with a history of psychic depression should be carefully observed and OCs discontinued if the depression recurs during OC use.

Women requiring drugs listed in Table 14 and may require higher doses of OCs or may need to use other methods of contraception. Alternatively, use of other types of anti-depressants may be considered.

Switching patients to OCs with lower progestin doses relieves symptoms of sleepiness and depression not due to organic causes (see Table 6).

EMOTIONAL CHANGES

Clinical Information

Emotional changes may include excitability, feelings of unrest, nervousness, and irritability.

Causal Factors

Emotional upset often occurs premenstrually in ovulatory women. Symptoms may be due to the premenstrual fluid-retention syndrome caused by sodium and water retention. Depending on their associations with fluid retention, these symptoms may be the result of either excessive or insufficient estrogenic activity in OCs. Symptoms may also be due to low blood glucose levels.

Irritability associated with depression during OC use or after discontinuance of OCs may be due to vitamin B_6 deficiency (2).

Management

If symptoms are relieved by sugar intake, patients have hypoglycemia. If the diagnosis of hypoglycemia is confirmed, patients should be advised to eat low-sugar/high-protein diets and should be switched to OCs with lower progestational and androgenic activities (see Table 6).

In a placebo-controlled, double-blind, cross-over study, nervousness during the first cycle only was related to high-estrogen content OCs (3).

If nervousness and irritability occur both during the days active OCs are taken and during pill-free days or if they occur without accompanying edema at any time, patients may be switched to OCs with greater estrogenic activities that do not exceed 35 mcg of estrogen.

32.

If irritability is accompanied by edema during the days active OCs are taken, patients should be switched to OCs with lower estrogenic activities.

Monophasic OCs may be helpful for patients with mood swings.

Vitamin B_6 may be helpful, especially with accompanying depression.

LIBIDO CHANGES

Clinical Information

Common terms for libido are sex drive, sexual feelings, and sexual nature. A statistically significant decrease in libido has been reported in some OC users. Decreased libido occurs most often with high-progestin/high-estrogen OCs. High doses of progesterone are used to decrease libido in male sex offenders. An increase in libido has also been suggested to occur in some OC users.

Causal Factors

Libido is related to the effective amount of testosterone in the blood, most of which is bound to sex hormone-binding gonadotropin (SHBG). A decrease in libido may be due to:
- Suppression of ovarian testosterone production
- A direct action on the brain by progestin
- An increase in SHBG induced by estrogens.

An increase in libido may result from:
- A decrease in SHBG
- Inherent androgenic effects of some progestins
- Reduced anxiety about becoming pregnant.

Management

If decreased libido occurs, patients may be switched to OCs with lower estrogenic and progestational activities or with higher androgenic activities. If increased libido occurs and is a problem, patients may be switched to OCs with lower androgenic and higher progestational activities.

238

PSYCHIATRIC DISORDERS

Clinical Information

Large controlled studies have shown no difference between OC users and nonusers in incidences of most psychiatric disorders (4). The incidence of phobic neuroses is decreased with OC use, but this is believed to be due to self-selection by the patient (1).

In institutionalized patients accustomed to long-term drug regimens, compliance is high and OC use is an appropriate choice in the absence of risk factors. Compliance is difficult to ensure in outpatients; thus, injections, or IUDs may offer better contraception for these patients (5).

The availability of long-acting implants makes sterilization for mental incompetents unnecessary except in rare circumstances.

EPILEPSY

Approximately 1% of the population is afflicted with epilepsy (6). Clinical studies have not demonstrated an increase in epilepsy when OCs are used, however, epileptic seizures are related to estrogen and progestin levels during the normal menstrual cycle (7). Most anti-epileptic drugs decrease steroid concentration and, therefore, effectiveness of OCs. One exception to this is valproic acid. Many anti-epileptic drugs, including valproic acid, are teratogenic.

Intramuscular (IM) medroxyprogesterone acetate (MPA) has been shown to decrease the number of seizures (8).

Management

Patients with epilepsy may require higher doses of progestins. IM MPA may also be used. Valproic acid does not induce hepatic enzymes and is the drug of choice for epileptic women who need contraception; however, it is associated with an increased risk of spina bifida.

References for Section 32: Neuropsychological System

1. Royal College of General Practitioners. Oral contraceptives and health: An interim report from the oral contraception study of the Royal College of General Practitioners. New York: Pitman, 1974.

2. Wynn V: Vitamins and oral contraceptive use. Lancet 1975; 1:561–564.

3. Goldzieher Joseph W et al.: A placebo-controlled, double-blind, cross-over investigation of the side effects attributed to oral contraceptives. Fertil Steril 1971;22:609–623.

4. Vessey MP et al.: Oral contraception and serious psychiatric illness: Absence of an association. Br J Psychiatry 1985;146:45–49.

5. Jungers P, Dougados M, Pelissier C, et al.: Influence of oral contraceptive therapy on the activity of systemic lupus erythematosus. Arthritis Rheum 1982;25:618–623.

6. Hauser WA, Hesdorffer DC: Epilepsy: Frequency, Causes, and Consequences. New York: Demos Publications, 1990.

7. Bachstrom T: Epileptic seizures in women related to plasma estrogen and progesterone during the menstrual cycle. Acta Neurol Scand 1976;54:321–347.

8. Mattson RH, Cramer JA, Caldwell BV, Siconolfi BC: Treatment of seizures with medroxyprogesterone acetate: Preliminary report. Neurology 1984;34:1255–1258.

NOTES

SECTION 33:
MUSCULOSKELETAL SYSTEM

LEG PAIN, CRAMPS, AND SWELLING

Clinical Information

Bilateral leg cramps and swelling of the lower extremities often disappear spontaneously after the third cycle of OC use.

Unilateral leg swelling may be due to thrombophlebitis or venous thrombosis.

Signs of thrombosis include:
- An increase in size and warmth of the leg
- Pain on palpation and dorsiflexion of the foot
- A palpable cord.

A rapid increase in pain over a 24-hour period indicates probable thrombosis as a cause.

Pain in the chest and/or shortness of breath may indicate that a pulmonary embolus has occurred.

Causal Factors

Bilateral leg pain may be insignificant and the result of fluid retention, especially if accompanied by cramps. Fluid retention due to OC use may result from either the estrogen or the progestin/androgen component of the OC.

Bilateral leg pain may also result from venous dilatation due to the progestin.

Unilateral leg pain may be the result of thrombophlebitis or thrombosis.

Management

In all cases of leg pain, an examination must be performed to rule out thrombosis or thrombophlebitis.

OCs should be stopped until the cause of pain is determined. A diagnosis of thrombosis or thromboembolism is an absolute contraindication to further OC use (see Section 26).

Bilateral swelling due to fluid retention may be relieved by switching the patient to an OC with lower estrogenic and/or progestational/androgenic activities. A low-sodium diet may also reduce edema.

Bilateral leg pain associated with venous dilatation or varicose veins may be relieved by switching the patient to an OC with lower progestational activity. Bilateral leg cramps may also be relieved by an increase in calcium intake.

If swelling and pain persist, an alternative method of birth control should be considered.

RHEUMATOID ARTHRITIS

Rheumatoid arthritis may be reduced by OC use (1, 2, 3, 4, 5). In three studies, the incidence of rheumatoid arthritis in OC users was reduced by 50% and the risk in women who had ever used OCs was reduced by 60% (2, 6, 7). Other studies involving smaller numbers of patients were unable to confirm a protective effect against rheumatoid arthritis in OC users or former users (8, 9).

MUSCLE FUNCTION

OCs do not usually affect athletic performance but may decrease endurance (10).

BONE MASS

OCs increase vertebral bone calcium by about 1% per year of use in premenopausal women (11). Radial bone mass increases with high-estrogen OCs, and bone calcium turnover is retarded with a moderately androgenic OC (12, 13).

Ever use of OCs reduced hip fracture in post-menopausal women by 25% in one retrospective study (14). The effect was greatest (44%) for use of greater than 50 mcg estrogen and for use after age 40.

References for Section 33: Musculoskeletal System

1. Liang MH et al.: Oral estrogen use, menopausal status, and relationship to rheumatoid arthritis. Ann Rheum Dis 1984;43:115.

2. Linos A et al.: Rheumatoid arthritis and oral contraceptives. Lancet 1978;2:871.

3. Royal College of General Practitioners Oral Contraceptive Study. Reduction in incidence of rheumatoid arthritis associated with oral contraceptives. Lancet 1978;1:569.

4. Vandenbroucke JP et al.: Noncontraceptive hormones and rheumatoid arthritis in premenopausal and postmenopausal women. JAMA 1986;255:1299.

5. Vandenbroucke JP et al.: Oral contraceptives and rheumatoid arthritis: Further evidence for a protective effect. Lancet 1982;2: 839–842.

6. Royal College of General Practitioners. Oral contraceptives and health: An interim report from the oral contraception study of the Royal College of General Practitioners. New York: Pitman, 1974.

7. Wingrave SJ, Kay CR: Reduction in incidence of rheumatoid arthritis associated with oral contraceptives. Lancet 1978;1:569.

8. Allebeck P et al.: Do oral contraceptives reduce the incidence of rheumatoid arthritis? Scand J Rheumatol 1984;13:140.

9. Del Junco DJ et al.: Do oral contraceptives prevent rheumatoid arthritis? JAMA 1985;254(14): 1938–1941.

10. Wirth JC, Lohman TG: The relationship of static muscle function to use of oral contraceptives. Med Sci in Sports Exerc 1982; 14:16.

11. Ory HW: Oral contraceptive use and breast diseases. In: Pharmacology of Steroid Contraceptive Drugs. Garattini S, Berendes HW (ed.) New York: Raven Press, 1977;179–183.

12. Chef R: Calcium metabolism during treatment with 2.5 mg Lyndiol®, a lynestrenol-mestranol combination. Bull Soc Roy Belg Gyn Ob 1966;36:473.

13. Rodin A et al.: Combined oral contraception and skeletal bone mass. Bone 1987;8:53.

14. Michaelsson Karl, Baron John A, Bahman Y Farahmand, Persson Ingemar, Ljunghall Sverker: Oral contraceptive use and risk of hip fracture: A case-control study. Lancet 1999; 1481–1484.

NOTES

SECTION 34:
INTEGUMENTARY SYSTEM

General

Complexion changes are a major concern of many women, especially teen agers. For the most part OCs cause an improvement in complexion. The estrogen component of OCs increases levels of SHBG and thereby removes free testosterone from the circulation (1, 2). Progesterone is an antagonist of testosterone and dihydrotesterone at the skin and hair follicle level. Estrogen and progesterone synergistically suppress ovarian secretion of testosterone, androstenedione, and DHEAS by inhibiting LH secretion.

HAIR GROWTH

Clinical Information

Excessive facial and body hair are ordinarily diminished in OC users because androgens of ovarian origin and serum free testosterone are suppressed during OC use. Hair loss (alopecia) is not related to OC use.

High androgen levels may cause an increase or darkening of facial and body hair.

Estrogens and natural progestin antagonize androgenic effects.

A 2003 randomized controlled study of the efficacy of 0.15 mg desogestrel plus 30 mcg EE (Desogen®) versus 0.15mg levonorgestrel plus 30 mcg EE (Nordette®) found that after 9 months both OCs caused a significant (33–36%) improvement in the Ferriman-Gallwey hirsuitism score (1). The level of SHBG was increased significantly in both groups but more so with Desogen. Ovarian androgen (androstenedione) was suppressed to a greater degree in the Nordette group. Despite these differences the clinical effect was nearly identical. Most OCs would be expected to have a similar beneficial effect on excessive hair growth.

Causal Factors

Most OCs are androgenic to some degree (see Table 6). Androgenic symptoms may result from:

- A decrease in sex hormone-binding globulin (SHBG) that may occur with some OCs with low estrogenic activities (3, 4)
- Failure to suppress endogenous ovarian androgen production
- Occupancy by progestin of androgen-binding sites on serum-binding globulins
- Inherent androgenic activity of a particular progestin.

A decrease in SHBG may occur with some OCs due to low estrogenic activities. This decrease allows increased circulating amounts of free androgen of adrenal or ovarian origin. Low estrogenic activity rather than high inherent androgenic activity is the probable cause of most androgenic symptoms if they begin during OC use.

Management

Alopecia, is not related to OC use and no change in dose or OC type is necessary. OCs with higher estrogen activity and or high progestin activity may be most effective in suppressing excessive hair growth (see Tables 6 and 9).

The rate of body hair growth should slow and sebum should be markedly decreased within one month following an effective switch in OCs. Actual loss of new body hair growth may take up to one year to occur.

If sebum production and body hair growth fail to decrease, patients should be evaluated for other causes of increased androgen, such as ovarian or adrenal tumor or hyperplasia.

34.

ACNE VULGARIS

Clinical Information

Acne is the result of increased sebum production associated with blocked and infected pores.

Causal Factors

Increased androgen levels cause increased sebum production, leading to pimples and acne. Abnormal circulating androgen levels are present in 90% of young women with acne. Testosterone, the most active androgen, is produced directly in the ovary and indirectly by peripheral conversion of weaker androgens produced by the adrenal glands.

Insulin resistance has recently been recognized as the cause of increased serum androgen levels and anovulation in women formerly thought to have polycystic ovarian syndrome.

Management

OCs with progestins that have low androgenic-to-progestin activity ratios (i.e., drospirenone, desogestrel, ethynodiol diacetate) and OCs with moderate-to-high estrogen contents are most likely to result in relief from acne and to block excessive hair growth. Ortho Tri-Cyclen®, a triphasic norgestimate OC containing 35 mcg EE, has received FDA approval for treatment of acne (5). However, other OCs containing the progestins listed above, especially when combined with higher estrogen doses, may be equally effective (2, 3, 6, 7) (see Tables 6 and 9). A 2003 randomized controlled study of the efficacy of 0.15 mg desogestrel plus 30 mcg EE (Desogen®) versus 0.15mg levonorgestrel plus 30 mcg EE (Nordette®) found that after 9 months mean acne lesion counts decreased by 58% for Desogen and by 53% for Nordette. The difference between the two OCs in improvement was not significant.

Androgenic symptoms that first appear after starting OCs are more likely to be due to low estrogen activity than to high androgenic activity of the progestin.

Diet changes and diligent cleansing of the skin will frequently result in relief of acne.

CHLOASMA

Clinical Information

Chloasma, also referred to as hyperpigmentation or mask of pregnancy, is a benign condition characterized by the appearance on the skin of brown patches of irregular shapes and sizes.

Chloasma occurs more frequently in women exposed to excessive sunlight, who normally have dark complexions.

Causal Factors

The cause of chloasma is unknown, but it may be related to increased melanocyte-stimulating hormone (melatonin) and to the progestational component of OCs. In a comparative trial of OCs containing norethindrone or NG and equal amounts of estrogens, the latter, which has higher androgenic and progestational potencies, was associated with a higher incidence of chloasma (8).

Management

Chloasma must be distinguished from other causes of hyperpigmentation, such as adrenal failure (Addison's disease). A switch to an OC with lower progestational and estrogenic doses and activities often results in a decrease in pigmentation (see Tables 5 and 6), though the pigmentation may never entirely disappear.

MELANOMA

A report of a possible 1.7 to 1.8 increased relative risk of melanoma in OC users (9) has not been confirmed. Three subsequent reports involving 612 women found no relationship between OC use and melanoma in the U.S. (10), Australia (11), or western Canada (12). These reports also found no relationship between melanoma and estrogen replacement but did find a significantly decreased incidence of melanoma in women who had experienced five or more births and in women who had undergone bilateral oophorectomy.

RASH AND ITCHING

Clinical Information

Symptoms of rash and itching, also referred to as pruritis, may be associated with:

- Skin eruptions
- Urticaria
- Exanthema.

Rashes and itching are common complaints and may be due to many causes other than OCs, including insect bites and contact dermatitis.

Causal Factors

Rash and itching may occur in women who are allergic to the inactive ingredients in OCs (e.g., lactose) or to dyes used to add color (see Table 5 for a list of inactive ingredients).

Rash or itching due to drug idiosyncrasy occurs in a small percentage of OC users as with any drug, and is usually due to the progestin component.

Management

Symptoms of rash and itching may indicate an underlying pathological condition, such as cholestatic jaundice or hepatitis (see Section 29).

If rash and itching are due to OC use, they may be due to either inactive ingredients or the progestin component. Patients may experience relief by switching to OCs with different inactive ingredients or different progestins (see Table 5).

LUPUS ERYTHEMATOSUS

Systemic lupus erythematosus is a relative contraindication for use of estrogen-containing OCs (13). Estrogen may cause cutaneous lupus to progress to systemic lupus by promoting B-cell hyper-responsiveness and inducing or increasing autoimmunity (14).

Women with from longstanding refractory lupus who are taking OCs may show significant symptomatic improvement and greater treatment responsiveness if they discontinue combination and multiphasic OC use (14).

Testosterone use may improve lupus symptoms. Pro-gestin-only OCs containing NG may be safely used by patients with lupus erythematosus.

TELANGIECTASIAS

Clinical Information

Telangiectasias (liver spots or spider nevi) are characterized by a central vessel that may be seen when a glass slide is placed over the lesion. These are usually found in the upper part of the body.

Causal Factors

Telangiectasias are due to capillary dilatation and fragility and occur more frequently with age.

Spider nevi may occur with cirrhosis of the liver. Telangiectasias that occur with OC use are thought to be related to estrogen.

Telangiectasias may be a manifestation of generalized purpura or of a hematological disorder.

Management

When telangiectasias are of recent origin and are not associated with evidence of bleeding elsewhere (such as in joints and extremities), they may be due to excess estrogenic activity. In such cases, patients should be switched to OCs with lower estrogenic activities.

References for Section 34: Integumentary System

1. Breitkopt DM, Rosen MP, Young SL, Nagmani M. Efficacy of second versus third generation oral contraceptives in the treatment of hirsuitism. Contraception 2003;67:349–53.
2. Rosen MP, Breitkopt DM, Nagmani N. A randomized controlled trial of second-versus third-generation oral contraceptives in the treatment of acne vulgaris. Am J Obstet Gynecol 2003;188: 1158–60.
3. Cullberg G et al.: Effects of a low-dose desogestrel/ EE combination on hirsutism, androgens, and sex hormone-binding globulin

in women with polycystic ovary syndrome. Acta Obstet Gynecol Scand 1985;64(3):195–202.

4. Wild RA et al.: Hirsutism: Metabolic effects of two commonly used oral contraceptives and spironolactone. Contraception 1991;44:113–124.

5. Redmond GP, Olson WH, Lippman JS, Kafrissen ME, Jones TM, Jorizzo JL: Norgestimate and EE in the treatment of acne vulgaris: A randomized, placebo controlled trial. Obstet Gynecol 1997;89:615–622.

6. Palatsi R, Hirvensalo E, Liukko P, et al.: Serum total and unbound testosterone and sex hormone binding globulin (SHBG) in female acne patients treated with two different oral contraceptives. Acta Derm Venereol (Stockh) 1984;64(6):517–523.

7. Pye RJ et al.: Effect of oral contraceptives on sebum excretion rate. Br Med J 1977;2:1581–1582.

8. Sanhueza H et al.: A randomized double-blind study of two oral contraceptives. Contraception 1979;20:29.

9. Walnut Creek Contraceptive Drug Study. Results of the Walnut Creek Contraceptive Drug Study. J Repro Med 1980;25(suppl):346.

10. Helmrich SP et al.: Lack of an elevated risk of malignant melanoma in relation to oral contraceptive use. J N Clin 1984;72(3): 617–620.

11. Green A, Bain C: Hormonal factors and melanoma in women. Med J Aust 1985;142(8):446–448.

12. Gallagher RP et al.: Reproductive factors, oral contraceptives, and risk of malignant melanoma: Western Canada Melanoma Study. Br J Cancer 1985;52(6):901–907.

13. Jungers P, Dougados M, Pelissier C, et al.: Influence of oral contraceptive therapy on the activity of systemic lupus erythematosus. Arthritis Rheum 1982;25:618–623.

14. Goldman EL: Estrogen OCs accelerate lupus progression. Obstet Gynecol News, 1997;14. 224 225

NOTES

SECTION 35: NUTRITIONAL AND WEIGHT CHANGES

NUTRITIONAL CHANGES

OCs may decrease serum levels of:
- Folacin (folic acid)*
- Pyridoxine (vitamin B_6)
- Riboflavin (vitamin B_2)
- Cobalamin (vitamin B_{12})
- Thiamine (vitamin B_1)
- Ascorbic acid (vitamin C)
- Calcitriol (vitamin D)
- Tocopherol (Vitamin E)
- Zinc
- Magnesium.

*One study found increased levels (1, 2)

Routine use of multivitamin supplements is usually unnecessary for OC users. Low levels of vitamin B_6, however, can cause depression and impaired glucose tolerance, a loss that can be adequately corrected by daily supplementation of 10 mg vitamin B_6.

In a study that measured folic acid, retinol (vitamin A), thiamine (vitamin B_1), riboflavin (vitamin B_2), pyridoxine (vitamin B_6), cyanocobalamin (vitamin B_{12}), tocopherol (vitamin E), carotenoids, and tryptophan in Thai women using OCs, the only significant findings were elevated vitamin A and folic acid.

Women who become pregnant soon after discontinuing OCs may have greater risks of folate deficiency. All women intending pregnancy, regardless of OC use, should begin taking neonatal vitamins containing folic acid three months prior to attempting conception in order to decrease the risks of neural tubal defects and other congenital anomalies that can result from folate deficiency.

Plasma levels of some nutrients (such as vitamin A, iron, and copper) increase with OC use. These increases are not substantial enough to cause clinical effects and may be beneficial for some women.

The clinical effects of severe vitamin and mineral deficiencies are shown in Table 13. Deficiencies marked enough to cause these symptoms are rare.

Causal Factors

Decreased intestinal absorption of vitamins and minerals causes many of the deficiencies associated with OC use. The most marked decreases are found in the water-soluble vitamins.

Pyridoxine is utilized in the metabolism of tryptophan. Because estrogen increases tryptophan production, more pyridoxine is needed for metabolizing the increased levels of tryptophan in OC users.

Estrogen also stimulates the metabolism of vitamins, resulting in decreased levels of some vitamins, especially B_2, B_{12}, C, in OC users.

Because estrogen increases vitamin A carrier protein in the blood, it is thought to be responsible for the increase in this fat-soluble vitamin in OC users.

Management

OC users who eat an adequate diet usually do not require vitamin supplementation unless they plan to become pregnant within three months. Table 13 lists dietary sources of important vitamins and minerals. Women who wish to increase their intakes of vitamins and minerals can do so by increasing their intakes of these source foods rather than by taking supplements.

WEIGHT INCREASE OR DECREASE

Clinical Information

Numerous studies have shown that as many women lose weight as gain weight while taking OCs. One study found that overweight women gained less weight than underweight women (3). Weight gain may actually be beneficial to poorly nourished women.

35

Causal Factors

Progestins, especially those with high androgenic activities, and estrogens can cause weight gain. Progestin- and/or androgen-induced weight gain may be due to:

- An anabolic effect, accompanied by increased appetite, OR
- An altered carbohydrate metabolism, which can cause hyperinsulinemia and is accompanied by symptoms of hypoglycemia.

Estrogen-induced weight gain is associated with an increase in subcutaneous fat, especially in the breasts, hips, and thighs, and is not accompanied by increased appetite.

Weight gain may also be associated with fluid retention due to either component of the OC. This type of weight gain is cyclic and is usually accompanied by other symptoms of fluid retention.

Management

OCs with lower progestational/androgenic activities may be of benefit if weight gain is accompanied by:

- Increased appetite
- Symptoms of hypoglycemia.

OCs with lower estrogenic activities may be of benefit if the weight gain:

- Occurs mainly in the breasts, hips, and thighs
- Is cyclic
- Is accompanied by bloating or edema.

CHANGES IN LABORATORY VALUES

Interactions with Laboratory Tests

OCs cause a number of laboratory changes, most of which are related to the estrogen component (see Table 10).

References for Section 35: Nutritional and Weight

1. Geurts TBP, Goorissen EM, Sitsen JMA: Summary of Drug Interactions with Oral Contraceptives, Parthenon Publishing Group, Carnforth UK, New York, 1993.

2. Wynn V: Vitamins and oral contraceptive use. Lancet 1975;1: 561–564.

3. Talwar PP, Berger GS: Side effects of drugs: The relation of body weight to side effects associated with oral contraceptives. Br Med J 1977;1:1637–1638.

ABBREVIATIONS

AFP	Alpha-fetoprotein
ASHD	Atherosclerotic heart disease
BBT	Basal body temperature
BTB	Breakthrough bleeding
CEE	Conjugated equine estrogen
CI	Confidence interval
CNS	Central nervous system
CVA	Cerebrovascular accident
CSBG	Cortecosteroid sex-binding globulin
CVD	Cardiovascular disease
DHEA	Dehydroeplandrosterone
DMPA	Depomedroxyprogesterone acetate
DS	Desogestrel
EC	Estradiol cypionate
ED	Ethinodial diacetate
EE	Ethinyl estradiol
GS	Gestodene
HDL-C	High-density lipoprotein cholesterol
IDD	Insulin-dependent diabetes
LDL-C	Low-density lipoprotein cholesterol
LNG	Levonorgestrel
MI	Myocardial infarction
MPA	Medroxyprogesterone actetate
NDA	New drug application (to FDA)
NE	Norethindrone
NEA	Norethindrone acetate
NET	Norethindrone enanthanate
NG	Norgestrel
NS	Norgestimate
OC	Oral contraceptive
OR	Odds ratio
RCGP	Royal College of General Practitioners
RCOG	Royal College of Obstetrics and Gynecology
RR	Relative risk
VTE	Venous thromboembolism
WHO	World Health Organization
WYS	Women years

Pharmaceutical Manufacturer References

Barr Laboratories, Inc.
400 Chestnut Ridge Road
Woodcliff Lake, NJ 07677
800-222-0190

Berlex Laboratories
300 Fairfield Road
Wayne, NJ 07470
973-694-4100

Duramed Pharmaceuticals, Inc.
5040 Lester Road
Cincinnati, OH 45213
800-222-0190

Monarch Pharmaceuticals
501 Fifth St.
Bristol, TN 37620
Direct Inquiries 800-776-3637

Organon, Inc.
375 Mt. Pleasant Ave.
West Orange, NJ 07052
Direct Inquiries 973-325-4500

Ortho-McNeil Pharmaceutical
Raritan, NJ 08869-0602
Medical Information 800-682-6532

Parke Davis
A Warner-Lambert Division
A Pfizer Company
201 Tabor Road
Morris Plains, NJ 07950
Customer Service 800-223-0432

Roberts Pharmaceutical Corp.
4 Industrial Way West
Eatontown, NJ 07724
Direct Inquiries 800-536-7878

Searle
100 Route 206 North
Peapack, NJ 07977
Direct Inquiries 888-768-5501

Warner Chilcott Laboratories
Rockaway 80 Corporate Center
100 Enterprise Drive, Ste. 280
Rockaway, NJ 07866
Direct Inquiries 800-521-8813

Watson Laboratories, Inc.
311 Bonnie Circle
Corona, CA
Customer Service 800-272-5525

Wyeth-Ayerst Pharmaceuticals
Division of American Home Products Corp.
PO Box 8299
Philadelphia, PA 19101
Direct General Inquiries 610-688-4400
Medical Info: Medical Affairs 800-934-5556

SECTION #36: INDEX

36.